meals

ALSO BY ANNABEL KARMEL

The Healthy Baby Meal Planner

favorite family meals

Annabel Karmel

ATRIA BOOKS

New York London Toronto Sydney

For my children, Nicholas, Lara, and Scarlett,
a constant source of inspiration

ATRIA BOOKS

1230 Avenue of the Americas
New York, NY 10020

Text copyright © 1999, 2005 by Annabel Karmel
Photographs copyright © 1999 by David Pangbourne and copyright © 2005 by Dave King

Originally published in Great Britain in 1999 as *Family Meal Planner* by Ebury Press

Published by arrangement with Cooking for Children Limited

Library of Congress Cataloging-in-Publication Data

Karmel, Annabel.
    [Family meal planner]
    Favorite family meals / Annabel Karmel.
        p.   cm.
    Originally published in Britain in 1999 as Family meal planner by Ebury Press.
    1. Cookery.   I. Title.

TX714.K3672 2006
641.5—dc22   2005055880

ISBN-13: 978-0-7432-7518-7
ISBN-10:   0-7432-7518-7

First Atria Books hardcover edition January 2006

10 9 8 7 6 5 4 3 2 1

ATRIA BOOKS is a trademark of Simon & Schuster, Inc.

Manufactured in the United States of America

For information regarding special discounts for bulk purchases,
please contact Simon & Schuster Special Sales:
1-800-456-6798 or business@simonandschuster.com.

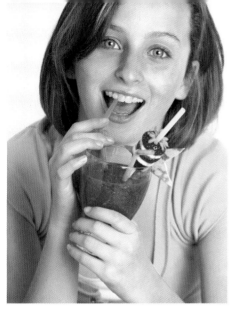

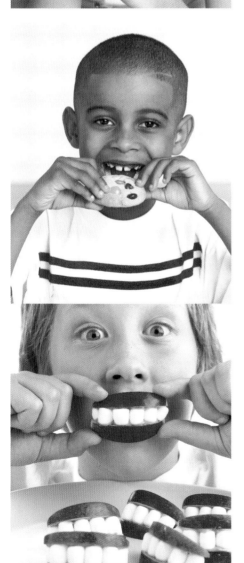

Contents

Introduction

This book will take the worry out of every-day cooking, because with it alongside you, you will know that you'll always have something in the house that can be made into a tasty meal for the family. These are some of my favorite tried and tested recipes for all occasions, from healthy breakfasts to lunch boxes, family suppers, recipes for entertaining, and even fun foods for children to cook themselves. As a busy mother of three children, I know how difficult it can be to find the time to make a home-cooked meal, so I have tried to create recipes that are quick and easy to prepare, healthy, and, of course, tasty. Each recipe has been tested on a panel of children who, naturally, didn't care how healthy the food was and were only impressed if it tasted good.

For many children, convenience and junk foods are no longer occasional foods but are becoming a regular part of their diet, and in this age of instant gratification, fewer and fewer families are sitting down to meals together. With the proliferation of processed packaged foods, many meals emanate from the freezer to be cooked in the microwave, and the kitchen is fast becoming the coldest room in the house. Healthy eating for children is crucial as it often sets the dietary pattern for life, and eating healthily from a young age can reduce the risk of developing diet-related diseases such as heart disease and some forms of cancer. For fighting disease, food is still the best medicine.

Food is more than just a biological need; its preparation expresses parental love and caring, and it's so very satisfying to see your family enjoy your lovingly prepared home-cooked meals. There was once a time when children ate mostly the same foods as their parents, and this book aims to provide you with recipes that the whole family will enjoy together. You don't need to be a Supercook. These recipes don't require split-second timing, special skills, or expensive equipment, and most of them can be prepared in less than 30 minutes.

Some weeks you'll be able to plan ahead and know what you're going to feed the family for supper on Friday when it's still only Monday, and other weeks you may only have time to think about Friday's dinner on Friday.

A bit of time spent planning, cooking ahead, and freezing some meals over the weekend will make the week ahead much more manageable. Decide on the week's meals and what advance cooking you need to do over the weekend. Then make a shopping list for the week and jot down on a calendar the fresh ingredients you will need to pick up during the week. Naturally, there will be weekends when you're too busy or the weather is too nice to spend time in the kitchen and so you can just plan simple meals for the week ahead such as Teriyaki Chicken Skewers (page 55) and salad and fresh fruit. There will also be occasions when you haven't even had time to do the shopping and it's already six o'clock, but you don't need to panic since there are lots of ideas here for delicious recipes that can be made from basic ingredients.

Rather than thinking what are we going to eat and what are the children going to eat, we should be thinking of one meal for the whole family. A good solution to the problem of family members who want meals at different times of the day is to freeze some food in individual portion sizes so that you have your own stock of healthy convenience foods that can be heated in the microwave in a matter of minutes. Very often when you are making a recipe it takes very little extra time to prepare more than you need so you have portions left over to freeze.

International cuisine can be another source of inspiration—perhaps make a Chinese dinner for the family, choosing some of the delicious, easy to prepare Chinese-style recipes such as Super Vegetarian Spring Rolls (page 124) followed by Chinese Noodles with Shrimp and Bean Sprouts (page 102) and lychees with Caramelized Almond Ice Cream (page 158) for dessert. Wouldn't it be fun to eat the food with chopsticks—you can buy child-friendly plastic chopsticks that are joined at the top, which makes it very easy for children to use.

This is a book of everyday family eating, and I hope it will be well thumbed and splattered with food and will help busy lifestyles become less chaotic. My aim is that this book will put the joy back into cooking, which is, after all, a labor of love.

Annabel Karmel

Organization

It's getting late, you've got work to finish for the next day, the phone keeps ringing, the children want help with their homework, and you haven't even thought about what you can make for supper. Do you find yourself staring at the contents of your cupboard for inspiration? Well, here's the answer to your problems.

First of all, here's a list of ingredients to stock in your kitchen so that you will always be able to rustle up a delicious meal for the family, and second, lots of recipes that can be frozen ahead. It takes very little extra effort or time to cook more than you need and freeze extra portions so you always have tasty, healthy dishes on hand, which can be defrosted and cooked at your convenience.

Coming up with varied meals can't always be done at the last minute. It's a good idea to work out what you will make three to four days in advance, write a list, and buy all the fresh ingredients that you don't already keep in your kitchen from the supermarket. With Internet shopping, you don't even need to leave home and it's a good idea to plan in advance.

Remember that it's easy to make more than you need when cooking a recipe and freeze extra portions so that you don't have to cook every day.

THE HEALTHY PANTRY

The key to making your life easier when it comes to planning weekly menus is stocking your kitchen with good basic ingredients. I have put together lists of the foods you need to try to keep in stock, basing them on the recipes in this book. Don't feel that you have to buy everything at once, and you can simply choose a selection of recipes that you would like to prepare and just buy the ingredients for those recipes.

Dry foods
Bread
Rice: basmati, long grain, and brown rice
Flour: whole wheat, all-purpose, self-rising
Cornstarch, white
Baking soda
Baking powder
Active dry yeast
Pasta: penne, tagliatelle, spaghettini, macaroni, lasagne, Chinese egg noodles
Sugar: superfine sugar, light brown sugar
Breakfast cereal: oatmeal, muesli, wheat germ, etc.
Dried fruit: apricots, raisins
Nuts: ground almonds, pecans, peanuts
Grains that don't take long to prepare: couscous, bulgur wheat
Split red lentils, green lentils
Desiccated coconut
Good-quality plain and white chocolate
Cocoa powder
Nonfat dry milk

Coconut milk
Tomato puree
Good-quality ready-made tomato sauce
Sun-dried tomatoes
Peanut butter
Maple syrup, honey
Sardines
Tuna fish in oil or water
Condensed cream of tomato soup
Condensed cream of mushroom soup
Condensed milk
Evaporated milk
Mandarin oranges
Peaches

Dried herbs and ground spices
Mixed dried herbs, basil, bay leaves, oregano, thyme, marjoram, paprika, turmeric, cumin, chili powder, blades of mace, nutmeg, black peppercorns, cinnamon, curry powder, ground ginger

Canned produce and jars
Chopped plum tomatoes
Corn
Baked beans

Fruit and vegetables
Variety of fruit
Salad vegetables
Onions

Garlic
Fresh gingerroot

Sauces, oils, and seasonings
Olive oil, sunflower oil, vegetable oil,
    sesame oil
Red wine vinegar, balsamic vinegar, rice
    wine vinegar (may find in Asian
    food section of store), cider vinegar,
    malt vinegar
Soy sauce
Oyster sauce
Worcestershire sauce
Tomato puree
Tomato sauce
Red pesto
Hoisin sauce
Salad dressing
Mayonnaise
Honey
Maple syrup
Curry powder
Ground mustard
Dijon mustard
Chicken stock and vegetable stock
    cubes or cans of stock
Sesame seeds
Pure vanilla extract
Lemon juice

Alcohol
Dry white wine
Sake (rice wine)
Mirin (sweet sake for cooking)
Sherry

IN THE REFRIGERATOR

To obtain the longest life possible from perishable foods, it would be a good idea to wash and tidy your refrigerator once a week.

Dairy and cooked foods should be stored at the top of the refrigerator with raw meats below in a sealed container.

Butter
Soft margarine
Low-fat plain yogurt
Cheddar cheese
Swiss cheese
Edam cheese
Parmesan cheese
Cream cheese
Eggs
Milk
Ready-made pudding

IN THE FREEZER

It's a good idea to freeze bread and butter for emergencies. It's also good to keep some ready-made frozen foods such as pizza or breaded chicken or fish in the freezer.

Frozen peas
Frozen spinach
Frozen corn
Frozen low-fat oven fries
Frozen pizza
Frozen boneless, skinless chicken
    breasts
Fish fillets with or without
    bread crumbs
Lean chopped meat
Lamb chops
Good-quality ice cream
Frozen raspberries

If you are buying fish or chicken in bread crumbs or batter, choose larger-portion sizes, as there will be less coating in proportion to the fish or chicken.

Buy thick-cut oven fries ("steak fries")—the thicker they are, the less fat they contain.

TIP
Keep a shopping list in the kitchen and have a house rule that whoever uses up the last of something adds the item to the list.

The Food Pyramid

Eating a balanced diet is all to do with choosing the right foods and eating them in the right proportions. For most of us that will mean eating more bread, cereals, starchy foods such as potatoes, pasta, and rice and more fruits and vegetables. This is the type of diet that adults and children over five should be eating.

Children under five need a diet higher in fat and lower in fiber because of their high energy requirements, and unlike their parents, they are also growing. Gradually, their diet will change to become more in line with that of an adult, lower in fat, particularly saturated fat, and higher in fiber. It is helpful to think of food groups rather than individual foods. The foods at the bottom of the pyramid are the ones we should be eating more of, and we should aim to eat less food from the food groups near the top.

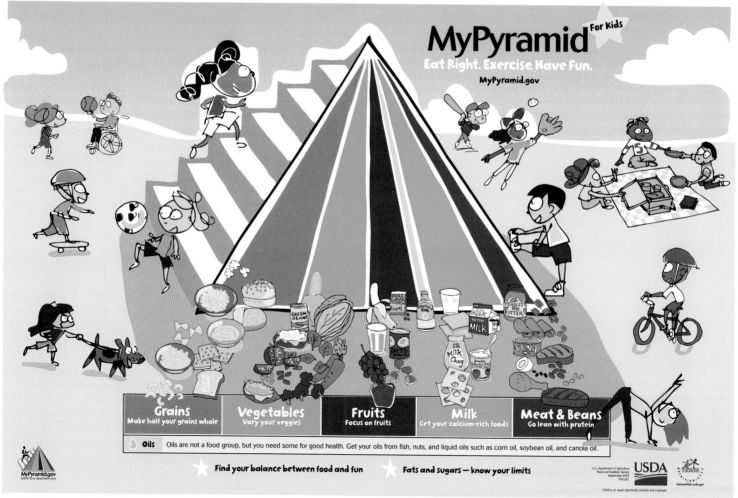

A balanced diet should contain approximately 20 percent protein, 35 percent fat, and 45 percent carbohydrates.

CARBOHYDRATES

These are the body's main source of energy and also provide vitamins, minerals, and fiber. Bread, pasta, potatoes, and rice can be used as the basis for many quick, healthy meals. Many people believe starchy foods such as bread and potatoes are high in calories, but this is not true. Plain boiled new potatoes are not fattening, but adding lots of butter to a baked potato can double its calorie content. A slice of bread contains about 65 calories, but buttering it increases this to 142 calories and spreading jam on top adds another 39 calories. Of course, this is less important for children who need more fat in their diet under the age of five, unless they are overweight. Whole-grain cereals and breads boost your intake of iron, vitamins, and fiber.

There are two types of carbohydrates: sugars and starches. In both types there are two forms again.

Sugars: natural fruits and vegetables,
refined sugars and honey, soft drinks, cakes, cookies, jam, desserts.

Starches: *Complex carbohydrates:* whole-grain breakfast cereal, whole-grain bread and flour, brown rice, potatoes, peas, bananas, and many other fruits and vegetables.
Refined carbohydrates: processed breakfast cereals, white flour, bread and pasta, white rice, cookies and cakes.

It is the complex carbohydrates and natural sugars that should form at least 50 percent of the calories in your diet.

Refined carbohydrates such as white bread and processed sweet breakfast cereals have lost many of their valuable nutrients during processing. Eat more complex carbohydrates; these energy-rich foods keep your blood sugar level constant because they release their sugar content into the bloodstream slowly. They also retain their vitamins and minerals and contain fiber, which encourages the elimination of toxins in the body.
See Vitamins on page xv for information on fruits and vegetables.

PROTEIN

It is reassuring to know that protein deficiency is almost unheard of in this country and most of us eat more protein than we need. Protein is essential for growth and repair of body tissue, and an inadequate supply of protein can lower resistance to disease and infection. The major protein foods are meat, chicken, fish, eggs, dairy products, beans, and lentils. It is good to serve one of these foods for lunch and supper. It's also quite likely that you might serve protein foods such as cheese or eggs at breakfast, too. Protein should make up 15 to 20 percent of your daily diet.

As a rough guide, eat meat or chicken three to four times a week, and it is recommended that two portions of fish are eaten each week, one of which should be an oily variety such as mackerel, tuna, salmon, or sardines. These and other oily fish are high in omega-3 fatty acids, which help lower blood pressure, and there is evidence that these fatty acids may help to protect against heart disease and strokes. Sardines are also a good source of bone-strengthening calcium and vitamin B_{12}. *See Brain-Boosting Foods on page xii on the importance of essential fatty acids for brain function.*

FOODS CONTAINING FAT; FOODS CONTAINING SUGAR

Potato chips, cakes, cookies, sweets, and soft drinks fall into this group. Since they often contain large quantities of fat, sugar, and salt, they should only be eaten occasionally and in small amounts. For adults and children over five, fat should provide no more than 35 percent of their total calorie intake. The way to achieve this is to cut down on junk food, cakes, and cookies. However, it's not realistic to ban these types of food altogether and they are perfectly fine as occasional foods or part of a meal.

Fats in moderation are an essential part of our diet. Fat makes food more palatable and plays an important role in providing energy, particularly in the diets of young children. It also facilitates the absorption of the fat-soluble vitamins A, D, E, and K. Vegetable oils and fish provide the essential fatty acids that the body cannot manufacture from other constituents in the diet.

There are two types of fat: saturated and unsaturated. Saturated fat is derived mainly from animal sources (meat, butter, cheese, eggs, and margarine), and unsaturated fat comes from vegetable sources (olive oil, sunflower oil, polyunsaturated margarine, and oily fish such as mackerel). We all need a certain amount of fat in our diet, but it is the type of fat that is important. Saturated fats can increase blood cholesterol levels and high intakes are linked to heart disease. It is a good idea to choose lean meats and vegetable oils for frying rather than butter. Cheese contains saturated fat; it is also a good source of calcium, protein, and vitamins.

FIVE PORTIONS A DAY

Health experts recommend that we should try to include five portions of fruit and vegetables in our diet every day. This helps to protect against cancers and heart disease and provides the right balance of vitamins, minerals, and fiber. As well as providing vitamins and minerals, fruit and vegetables also contain many other biologically active substances called phytochemicals. There is growing scientific evidence for the anti-cancer effects of the five hundred phytochemicals identified so far and there may be thousands more.

Different fruits and vegetables contain different vitamins and minerals, so try to include as much variety as you can. Fruits, vegetables, and juice high in vitamin C help iron to be absorbed from other foods, so ensure that you and your family eat some at each meal. Also fruit and vegetables are low in fat and calories and provide a natural source of fiber, which helps to keep the digestive system in order. Vitamin supplements contain only a small proportion of the benefits available in fruits and vegetables themselves.

BRAIN-BOOSTING FOODS

Don't let your child skip breakfast. Numerous studies have shown that a high-fiber breakfast—muesli, hot cereal, whole-grain cereal, or toast—helps to ensure a steady supply of blood sugar for long-lasting energy and good concentration. Sugary refined cereals and white bread are broken down quickly, rapidly releasing sugar in the blood. This gives a quick burst of energy followed by a drop in sugar levels, leaving a child tired, unable to concentrate, and hungry.

Iron deficiency is the most common nutritional deficiency in developed countries. Two of the main symptoms are tiredness and lack of concentration, so increasing iron intake could well improve your child's schoolwork as well as health. Iron is important for transporting oxygen in the blood to all organs in the body, including the brain; therefore, iron is important for good brain function. Red meat provides the best source of iron (see page xiv).

Oily fish rich in omega-3 fatty acids are important for brain function and concentration, so try to give children fish such as fresh tuna, salmon, sardines, or mackerel twice a week or buy omega-3-enhanced eggs, which are rich in fatty acids. Some hyperactive children are deficient in essential fatty acids and it is worthwhile having them tested, as research suggests that taking a 1,000 mg supplement of omega oils can help improve concentration in children who have attention deficit disorders and can also help with some motor learning difficulties.

Keeping hydrated helps the brain function at its best, so make sure your child drinks plenty of water. Children need about a quart of water a day.

HOW TO CHOOSE A HEALTHY DIET

Foods	Choose more often	Choose less often
Meat, poultry, fish, shellfish, nuts, and seeds	Lean cuts of meat trimmed of fat, poultry without skin, fish and shellfish, lean luncheon meat, canned tuna, sardines, seeds, nuts.	Fatty cuts of meat, bacon, and sausage, organ meats, fried chicken, high-fat luncheon meat.
Eggs and dairy products	Natural yogurt, low-fat yogurt, and 1% or 2% milk for adults, low-fat cheese (cottage cheese, Edam, low-fat Cheddar), boiled or poached eggs.	Cream, full-fat cheese (for adults), fried eggs, processed cheese.
Fats and oils	Polyunsaturated fats such as margarine and sunflower, grapeseed, safflower, sesame, soy, rapeseed, canola, corn, and olive oils.	Saturated fats such as butter, lard, and margarine.
Breads, cereals, pasta, rice, lentils, beans, cookies, cakes	Whole-grain bread, whole-grain breakfast cereal, pasta, and rice, dried beans and lentils, baked goods made with unsaturated oil or margarine, plain cookies.	White bread, refined sugar-coated cereals, sugary cookies, cakes, croissants.
Vegetables	Fresh or frozen raw vegetables, salads, stir-fried vegetables, dark leafy greens, and deep yellow or orange vegetables are particularly good.	Fried vegetables (french fries, potato chips), vegetables cooked with a lot of butter (mashed potatoes).
Fruits	Fresh, frozen, canned, or dried fruit, pure fruit juice; eat a wide variety of fruits—citrus and berry fruits are particularly good.	Canned fruit in syrup, fruit juice with added sugar, creamy fruit desserts.
Sweet foods	Good-quality ice cream, frozen yogurt, fresh fruit pops, cereal-and-dried-fruit bars.	Candy, creamy desserts, chocolates, gelatin, sugary ice pops, soft drinks.

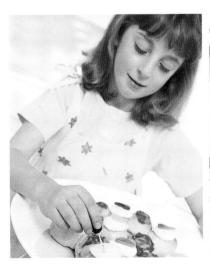 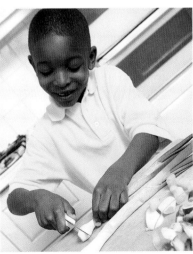 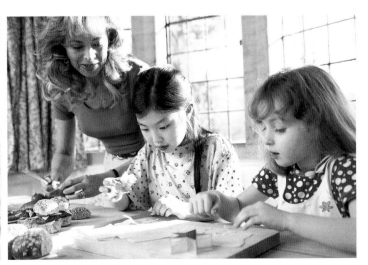

CALCIUM

Calcium is important for the health and formation of bones and teeth and is therefore particularly important for growing children. Calcium is also important for smooth functioning of the muscles, including the heart. Many teenagers are significantly deficient in calcium, which is vital to help build healthy bones during the teenage period of rapid growth. Between twelve and sixteen years for girls and thirteen and eighteen years for boys is a crucial period of bone and muscle growth.

Wheat bran, high-fiber cereals, and the tannin in tea and coffee can hinder the absorption of calcium. So if you drink tea or coffee, leave a sufficient gap before or after your meal.

Dairy foods provide the best source of calcium. Twelve ounces of milk a day or an equivalent such as yogurt, cheese, or milk puddings provides adequate calcium between the ages of one and five. Babies and young children should always be given whole milk and dairy products, as they contain essential nutrients for early growth.

Other moderately good sources: *dark green leafy vegetables, tofu, sardines, sesame seeds, and nuts.*

IRON

Iron deficiency is the most common nutritional problem in the developed world. Iron's main function is to carry oxygen from the lungs to all the cells in the body. Iron also helps to increase our resistance to infection and aids the healing process. Lack of adequate iron can lead to anemia, which will result in tiredness and lack of energy. Women, particularly teenage women, need to ensure there is enough iron in their diet, as it is lost in the blood during menstruation. Girls who are dieting and those who switch to a vegetarian diet are particularly at risk.

There are two types of iron—one is found in foods of animal origin such as red meat or oily fish and is easily absorbed by the body, and the other is found in foods of plant origin such as green vegetables or whole-grain cereals, and this is more difficult for the body to absorb. However, including a good source of vitamin C at the same meal, such as a glass of fresh orange juice or sliced kiwifruit and vegetables such as sweet bell pepper or cauliflower, will help to increase the absorption of iron in non-meat sources. Also, if meat or fish is eaten at the same meal as the plant type of iron, the iron is better absorbed.

By mixing lean meat with dark green leafy vegetables you can improve the absorption of iron from the vegetables by about three times. Since the richest and best-absorbed sources of iron are meats and meat products, vegetarians should be careful to ensure they include enough iron-rich foods and vitamin C in their daily diet. Tea, coffee, and bran reduce iron absorption.

Good sources: *red meat, particularly liver, oily fish (such as salmon, sardines, or mackerel), chicken or turkey (dark meat), lentils, baked beans, fortified breakfast cereals, bread, green leafy vegetables, dried fruit, especially apricots.*

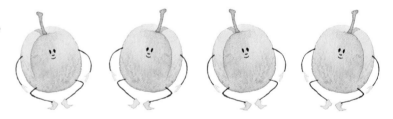

SMUGGLING EXTRA MILK

There are plenty of ways to add milk to other foods:

■ make fruit milk shakes

■ mash potatoes with plenty of milk

■ make dishes with cheese sauce, for example, cauliflower with cheese or macaroni with cheese

■ sprinkle grated cheese on pasta

■ offer yogurt

■ whip some half-set flavored gelatin with a can of evaporated milk

■ serve custard or good-quality ice cream with cake

Vitamins

There are two types of vitamins: water-soluble (B complex and C) or fat-soluble (A, D, E, and K). Water-soluble vitamins except for vitamin B_{12} cannot be stored in the body, so foods containing these should be eaten daily. They are destroyed by heat and dissolve in water, so foods containing these vitamins should not be overcooked. Fat-soluble vitamins are stored in the body, so excessive intake can be damaging.

Vitamin A
(Includes beta-carotene and retinol): important for growth, fighting infection, healthy skin and hair, strong bones, tooth enamel, and night vision.
Good sources of beta-carotene: *carrots, tomatoes, red pepper, apricots, mangoes, cantaloupe, sweet potato, dark green leafy vegetables.*
Good sources of retinol: *liver, cheese, eggs.*

B complex vitamins
Important for growth, development of a healthy nervous system, food digestion. No foods except liver and yeast extract contain all of the vitamins in the B group.
Good sources: *meat, eggs, sardines, tofu, dark green leafy vegetables, nuts, dairy products, whole-grain cereals, bananas.*

Vitamin C
Needed for growth and repair of body tissues, healthy skin, and healing of wounds. It is also important because it helps the body to absorb iron.
Good sources: *citrus fruit, strawberries, black currants, blackberries, kiwifruit, sweet pepper, dark green leafy vegetables, potatoes.*

All in a day's food
Any of the following provides a day's vitamin C intake for the average adult.

1 medium orange
1 medium mango
1 kiwifruit
1 grapefruit
2½ ounces raw cauliflower
¼ sweet red pepper, raw
1 medium glass freshly squeezed orange juice

Vitamin D
This is nicknamed the sunshine vitamin because it can be manufactured by the body when the skin is exposed to sunlight. It is needed to absorb calcium and posphorus for healthy bones and teeth.
Good sources: *salmon, tuna, sardines, milk and dairy products, eggs, margarine.*

Vitamin E
Necessary for the maintenance of the body's cell structure and helps the body to create and maintain red blood cells.
Good sources: *vegetable oils, wheat germ, nuts.*

VITAMIN C AND SMOKING
An average adult needs about 40 mg vitamin C per day. Smokers need up to three times as much because the chemicals from cigarettes destroy the vitamin.

HOME FREEZING OF COOKED FOODS

When you are preparing a recipe it takes only a little more effort to make enough for several meals. You can then serve part of the food freshly cooked and freeze the extra food in meal-size portions. Recipes in this book suitable for freezing are marked with a ❄.

■ Freeze food promptly as soon as it has cooled to room temperature.

■ Cool foods as quickly as possible before packaging—you can speed up the process by placing the container of food in a large pan of ice water.

■ Freeze and store foods at 0°F or less. It's a good idea to purchase a freezer thermometer that can withstand a wide range of temperatures and check the temperature of your freezer regularly.

■ Always reheat food until piping hot and then allow to cool down before eating in order to kill off any bacteria.

■ Slightly undercook prepared foods. They will finish cooking when reheated.

■ Never refreeze meals that have been frozen and never reheat more than once.

■ Bread wrappers are not sufficiently moisture-vapor resistant to be used for freezing. Use proper freezer bags instead.

■ Label and date all packages.

SALT

Children should have no more than about 4 g of salt a day but most eat twice as much. A high salt intake is linked to high blood pressure and heart disease, so try to limit the amount you add to food so that children don't develop a taste for it. Use herbs and spices to add flavor. About 75 percent of the salt we eat comes from processed foods and is also hidden in foods such as cereals, ketchup, and bread.

HOW TO READ FOOD LABELS

When buying processed foods always look carefully at the labels for the list of contents.

■ Choose foods that are low in sugar, salt, and saturated fat and do not contain monosodium glutamate, coloring, or artificial flavors.
■ Ingredients are listed in order of decreasing weight, so if sugar or saturated fat appear near the top of the list, you may want to think again before buying that product.
■ Sugars can be listed in a variety of guises, among them dextrose, glucose, fructose, and high fructose corn syrup.
■ Sweetening food with honey, concentrated fruit juice, or brown sugar is no better for your teeth than any other kind of sugar.
■ Often labels break carbohydrates into starch and sugars and it is useful to know that 4 grams of sugar equals 1 teaspoon.
■ Below is a chart to show acceptable content of fat, sugar, fiber, and sodium per serving.
■ Most labels give the amount of sodium in grams per 100 g of food. To convert sodium to salt multiply the amount by 2.5, for example, 1 g of sodium = 2.5 g of salt.

Per 100 grams/ 4-ounce serving	A lot	A little
Fat	20 g or more	2 g or less
Saturates	5 g or more	1 g or less
Sugars	10 g or more	2 g or less
Fiber	3 g or more	0.5 g or less
Sodium	0.5 g or more	0.1 g or less

(Approved by MAFF and the British Heart Foundation)

A Vegetarian Diet

More and more people are choosing to become vegetarian, and a vegetarian diet can be very healthy. However, it is important not to give up meat without replacing it with other sources of the nutrients that meat contains, particularly iron, protein, and B vitamins.

Animal proteins, including dairy products, contain all the amino acids that the body needs. However, soy is the only plant-based food that contains all the amino acids. In order to get a high-quality protein at each meal, you should try to include some dairy food or combine different non-animal proteins such as grains and legumes, which do not contain all the essential amino acids. There are many vegetarian recipes included in this book.

A healthy vegetarian diet should contain staple foods such as whole-grain bread, pasta, potatoes, and rice, lots of fresh fruits and vegetables, nuts, seeds, and legumes, and low-fat non-animal sources of protein, such as tofu, and low-fat dairy products. Take care not to eat too much high-fat dairy products and eggs.

Some teenage girls who start dieting and also choose to become vegetarian may cut out meat from their diet without replacing it with a suitable plant source of iron. This could cause problems, as they are particularly prone to iron deficiency due to the loss of blood as they start their periods (see Iron on page xiv for increasing the absorption of iron).

Vitamin B_{12} is vital for making DNA and is needed for the growth and division of cells. It is only found in foods of animal origin such as meat, poultry, fish, eggs, and dairy products. Some breakfast cereals are also fortified with vitamin B_{12}. Vegetarians can obtain sufficient vitamin B_{12} from eggs and dairy products, but vegans should take supplements or eat foods fortified with the vitamin.

NUTS

Small children can be allergic to a number of foods, particularly peanuts, sesame seeds, milk, eggs, wheat, soybeans, fish, and shellfish. Peanuts can trigger one of the worst allergic reactions— anaphylactic shock. The throat swells and breathing becomes difficult. In families with a history of any kind of food allergy, it is best to avoid all products containing peanuts until the child is three years old. If there is no allergic history, peanut butter can be used from six months. Because of the danger of inhalation, whole nuts should not be given to young children under five years of age.

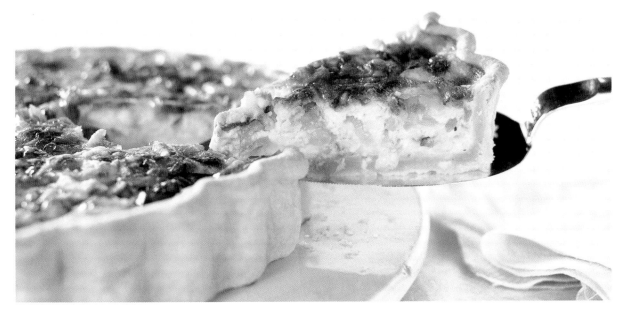

Caramelized Onion and Swiss Tart (see page 126)

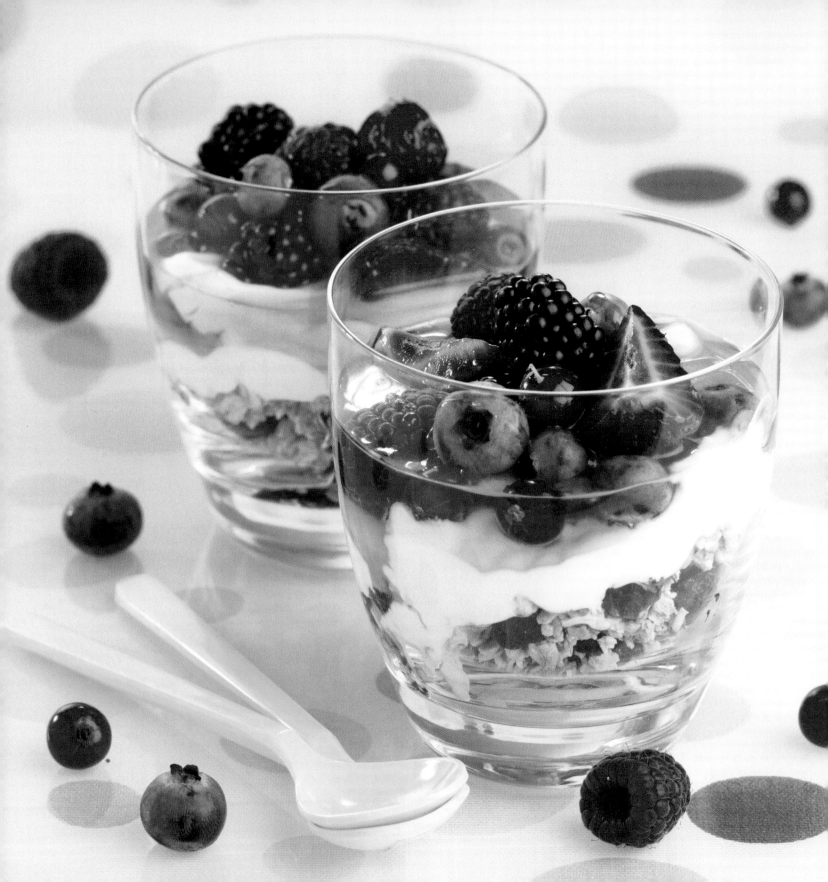

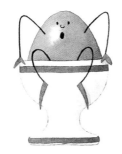

Breakfast
Suggestions

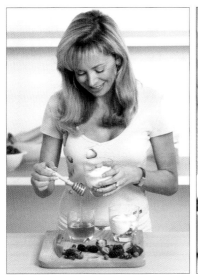
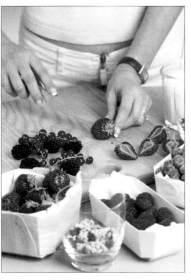
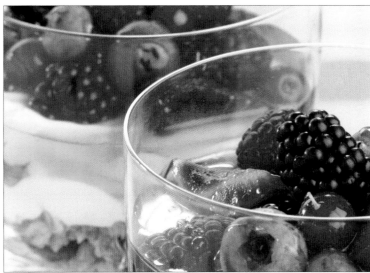

Breakfast Suggestions

The first meal of the day is also the most important. It will probably have been at least 12 hours since your last evening meal and blood sugar levels will be low. If you attempt to skip breakfast, then you may suffer various symptoms such as shakiness, headaches, and lack of concentration. You will probably then feel hungry later in the morning and crave something sweet, which is your body telling you that it needs glucose fast. It is much better, particularly for children who have high energy and nutrient requirements and who have a long morning at school ahead of them, to start the day with a balanced nutritious breakfast. Here's how to make sure that your child gets a good balanced nutritious breakfast.

FRUIT AND FRUIT JUICE

Choose a wide variety of seasonal fruits. Make fresh fruit salads or a mixture of berries served with yogurt and honey or prepare a colorful fruit plate. Berry and citrus fruits are particularly good in your child's diet. Breakfast should supply a good mix of starch and sugars. Sugar is best provided in the form of fruit or fruit juice, which is quickly broken down into glucose to raise energy levels as well as providing vitamin C, which helps to boost immunity.

BREAD, GRAINS, NUTS, AND SEEDS

The type of carbohydrates you give your child affects their energy level and their ability to concentrate. Unrefined carbohydrates such as oatmeal, muesli, and whole-grain bread get broken down slowly into sugar in the blood, providing a steady supply of energy, whereas sugary refined cereals and white bread give a quick burst of energy followed by a drop in sugar levels, leaving your child tired, unable to concentrate, and hungry. Adding extras such as sunflower and sesame seeds, chopped nuts, and dried fruit to cereals will boost their nutritional content.

The higher vitamin, mineral, and fiber content of whole-grain bread makes it the healthiest choice.

PROTEIN

Try to pick at least one calcium-rich protein food such as milk, yogurt, or cheese every day. Choose whole milk rather than low-fat varieties for children under five unless they are overweight. Eggs are an excellent source of protein and iron for your child and are very versatile.

Eggs should be served to young children with the white and yolk cooked until solid.

BREAKFAST CEREALS

A bowl of cereal is a healthy start to the day for your child, but you will need to choose carefully. Many of the cereals designed to appeal to children are highly refined and packed full of sugar (some contain almost 50 percent sugar). Ignore claims about added vitamins and minerals—vitamins are added to replace losses during processing. It is much better to choose whole-wheat cereals that are not coated in sugar such as oatmeal or muesli. Even if your child adds some sugar it will still be a lot less than the 4 to 5 teaspoons you might find in some cereals. Eating cereal also ensures that your children get milk, which provides both protein and calcium.

TIP
Very fresh eggs will contain fewer bacteria than older eggs, so try to find eggs that display the date.

Quick Breakfasts

FRUIT SALAD WITH HONEY YOGURT DRESSING

Make a fruit salad using seasonal fruits and top with a mixture of yogurt and honey. Alternatively, make a fruit plate and serve with a bowl of yogurt and honey for dipping.

STEWED FRUIT

Stewed fruit, such as cooking apple cooked with a little brown sugar and cinnamon or rhubarb with some fresh orange juice and brown sugar, makes a nice change for breakfast. Alternatively, make a baked apple with honey, raisins, and a teaspoon of butter and serve it cold for breakfast.

BREAKFAST CEREAL PLUS

Adding fresh fruits or dried fruits like chopped dried apricots to breakfast cereals will give sweetness without the need for sugar.

FUNNY SHAPE FRENCH TOAST

Lightly beat together 1 egg and 2 tablespoons of milk. Cut the bread into shapes using novelty cookie cutters, dip it into the egg mixture, and fry in butter until golden.

BOILED EGGS WITH SOLDIERS

Place the eggs in a saucepan, cover with cold water, and place on high heat. Bring to a boil and then reduce the heat to a simmer and cook for 4 to 5 minutes. Serve surrounded by fingers of toast, spread with a little butter. They are delicious dipped into the egg.

CRISPY BACON WITH TOMATO

Split and toast an English muffin. Top the cut sides with thinly sliced tomato, a little salt and pepper, and a pat of butter. Broil for 2 to 3 minutes, until the tomato softens. Top with crispy bacon.

TOAST WITH PEANUT BUTTER, HONEY, AND BANANAS

Spread slices of toasted whole-grain bread with peanut butter and a little honey and top with thinly sliced banana.

FRUITY MILK SHAKES

Blend together fresh fruit and milk to make delicious milk shakes. Try combinations such as fresh strawberries and banana, and peaches, nectarines, or fresh dates and banana. For a richer milk shake, add a refreshing scoop of ice cream.

SCRAMBLED EGGS PLUS

Make scrambled eggs extra special by adding ingredients such as chopped tomatoes, grated cheese, or ham. These should be added 1 minute before the eggs are done.

BREAKFAST SUNDAE

Into a sundae glass, spoon layers of yogurt, fresh fruit (such as mixed berries), and crunchy breakfast cereal until the glass is full.

Strawberry and Banana Yogurt Shake

Makes 1 tall glass

1 small banana, sliced
4 strawberries

2 tablespoons orange juice
½ cup vanilla yogurt

Put the banana, strawberries, and orange juice into a blender or food processor and puree. Add the yogurt and puree until smooth.

Perfect Oatmeal

A bowl of oatmeal makes a satisfying and nourishing breakfast and will help to keep energy levels up until lunchtime. The soluble fiber in oats also helps to lower blood cholesterol levels. These extras will make oatmeal taste even better: ready-made apple, apricot, or plum compote; maple syrup or honey; chopped banana and a little brown sugar; chopped dried fruit such as apricots; a chopped dessert apple, tossed in a pan with melted butter, brown sugar, and cinnamon.

Makes 2 bowls

1 cup rolled oats
2 cups milk (or water)

2 tablespoons strawberry jam
Blueberries or raspberries

Mix the oats with the milk or water in a saucepan. Bring to a boil and then simmer, stirring occasionally, for 5 minutes. Stir the strawberry jam in a bowl until it turns runny and then drizzle it in a spiral pattern onto the cereal. Add some blueberries to decorate the spiral pattern.

Muesli with Yogurt, Honey, and Fruit

Makes 1 serving

3 tablespoons muesli
½ cup plain yogurt
2 teaspoons honey

Fresh fruit, such as raspberries,
peaches, blueberries

Simply mix together the muesli, yogurt, and honey and top with the fresh fruit. Larger fruits such as strawberries or peaches are best cut into small pieces.

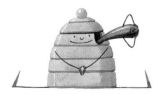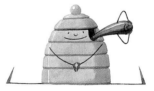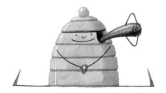

Best-Ever Banana Bread

This banana bread is wonderfully moist and is great for breakfast or lunch boxes. This keeps well, but you can also wrap slices in plastic wrap and freeze in plastic freezer bags. Many children aren't keen on nuts, so you can omit them from this recipe. Nut allergies are also a very real problem (see page xvii).

Makes 8 slices

1 stick butter
1 cup brown sugar
1 egg
1 pound bananas, mashed
3 tablespoons plain yogurt
1 teaspoon pure vanilla extract

1½ cups all-purpose flour
1 teaspoon baking soda
1 teaspoon ground cinnamon
¼ teaspoon salt
¾ cup raisins
2 tablespoons chopped pecans or walnuts (optional)

Preheat the oven to 350°F and grease and line an 8½ x 4¼ x 2½-inch loaf pan. Beat the butter and sugar together until creamy, then add the egg and continue to beat until smooth. Add the mashed bananas, yogurt, and vanilla.

Sift together the flour, baking soda, cinnamon, and salt and beat this gradually into the banana mixture. Finally, stir in the raisins and chopped nuts, if using. Bake for about 1 hour or until a toothpick inserted in the center comes out clean.

TIP

If time is short in the morning, get some of the breakfast organized the night before. Have cereal ready in bowls, perhaps prepare a muesli and keep it in the refrigerator overnight and simply stir in some fresh fruit in the morning, or bake some banana bread the day before and have it ready on the table. If your child is really rushed in the morning, let him take some portable food with him on the way to school such as a banana, home-baked muffins, or some dried apricots.

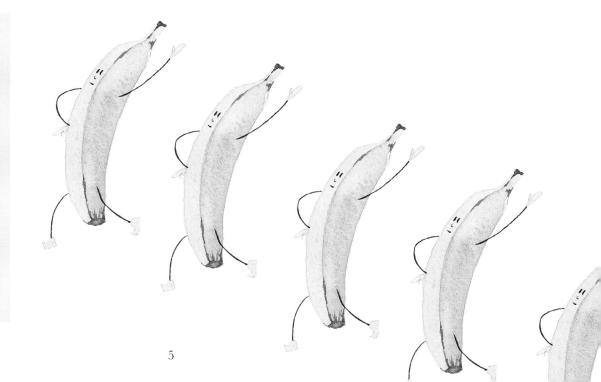

Cheesy Bread Shapes

These are good fun for children to make, as they love to knead the dough and mold it into animal shapes. On a cool morning, you might like to consider warming them in the oven before eating.

Makes 6 bread shapes

1½ cups all-purpose flour, plus flour to dust
1 teaspoon ground mustard
Pinch of salt
1½ teaspoons active dry yeast
3 cups warm water
½ teaspoon superfine sugar
1 teaspoon vegetable oil
½ cup grated Cheddar cheese
1 scallion, finely chopped

Decoration

1 egg, lightly beaten
Currants
Grated cheese
Sesame seeds
Poppy seeds

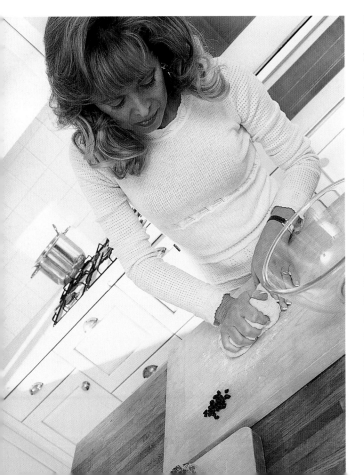

Sift the flour, mustard, and salt into a bowl. Place the yeast in a mixing bowl, pour in the warm water, stir in the sugar, and mix with a fork. Allow to stand until the yeast has dissolved and starts to foam, about 10 minutes. Stir in the oil and gradually mix in the flour mixture. If the dough is sticky, add a little extra flour. Transfer to a floured work surface and knead gently for about 5 minutes to make a smooth, pliable dough. Gradually knead the grated cheese and scallion into the dough to give it a streaky effect.

Shape the dough into rolls or animal shapes and put them onto a greased baking tray. Cover loosely with a kitchen towel and put them in a warm place to rise for about 1 hour or until doubled in size.

Preheat the oven to 400°F. Brush the shapes with the beaten egg and add currants for eyes. Sprinkle the tops with grated cheese, sesame seeds, or poppy seeds. Bake for 15 to 20 minutes or until golden. They are done if they sound hollow when tapped underneath. Transfer to a wire rack to cool.

 The "kids in the kitchen" symbol indicates where a recipe is suitable for children to make themselves.

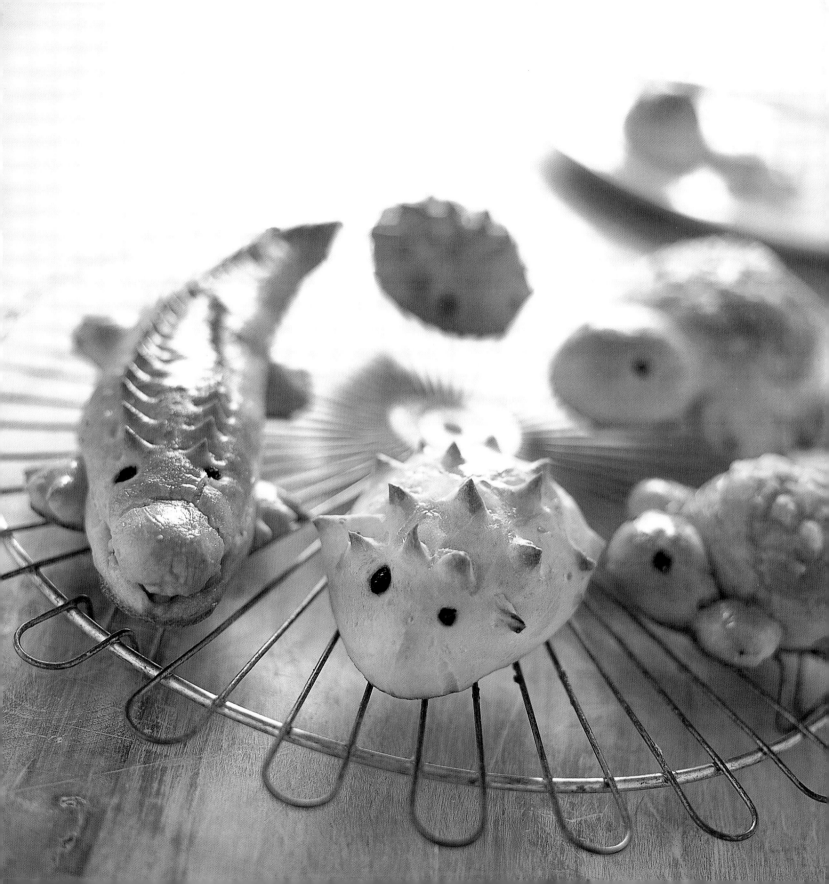

Welsh Rarebit

This is the perfect mixture for a really tasty Welsh rarebit. Traditionally, Welsh rarebit is flavored with beer, but you can use milk instead. To make fresh bread crumbs simply tear a slice of white bread into pieces and whizz in a food processor.

Makes 2 servings

1½ cups grated sharp Cheddar cheese
2 tablespoons milk (or beer if making for adults)
Few drops of Worcestershire sauce
Generous pinch of ground mustard

1 egg yolk, lightly beaten
3 tablespoons fresh white bread crumbs
2 thick slices whole-grain or white bread
Paprika, for sprinkling

Place the cheese and milk (or beer, if using) in a saucepan over low heat, stirring until melted. Add the Worcestershire sauce and mustard and stir in. Remove from the heat and beat in the egg yolk. Stir in the bread crumbs. Preheat the broiler. Toast the slices of bread and spread with the rarebit topping, then sprinkle with paprika. Cook the rarebits under the broiler until golden and bubbling, about 2 minutes.

Cheese, Chive, and Tomato Omelet

This is a delicious folded omelet, flavored with chives and filled with fresh tomatoes and melted cheese. If you don't have any chives, then make an herb omelet using ¼ teaspoon mixed dried herbs. Eggs are a good source of protein and are rich in vitamins and minerals.

Makes 1 serving

2 eggs
1½ teaspoons snipped fresh chives
Salt and freshly ground black pepper

1 tablespoon butter
2 tomatoes, peeled and roughly chopped
¼ cup grated Cheddar or Gruyère cheese

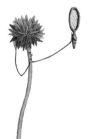 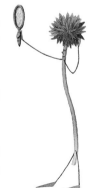

Beat the eggs with the chives and season with a little salt and freshly ground black pepper. Melt the butter in an 8-inch frying pan, add the beaten eggs and chives, and swirl the mixture around to coat the pan evenly.

When the edges of the eggs begin to set, lift the eggs with a spatula, tilt the pan toward the edge you have lifted, and let the uncooked eggs flow underneath the cooked portions.

Place the pan back on the burner. Spoon the tomatoes and grated cheese onto one side of the omelet. Fold over and cook for about 1 minute over gentle heat, until the omelet is set and the cheese is melted.

Perfect Pancakes

Pancakes for breakfast are a real treat and you can make delicious, really thin pancakes with this foolproof batter. Sprinkle them with lemon juice and dust with confectioners' sugar or serve with maple or light corn syrup and perhaps some fresh fruit. These pancakes can be made in advance, refrigerated, and then reheated just before serving. Pancakes also freeze very well. Interleave with nonstick baking paper, then wrap in foil, and freeze for up to a month. Thaw at room temperature for several hours.

Makes 12 pancakes

¾ cup all-purpose flour
Generous pinch of salt
2 eggs

1 cup milk
4 tablespoons melted butter

Sift the flour with a big pinch of salt into a mixing bowl, make a well in the center, and add the eggs. Use a balloon whisk to incorporate the eggs into the flour and gradually whisk in the milk. Stir the mixture until smooth, but do not overmix.

Use a heavy-bottomed 6- to 7-inch frying pan and brush with the melted butter (either use a pastry brush or dip some crumpled paper towel into the butter to coat the base of the pan) and when hot, pour in about 2 tablespoons of the batter. Quickly tilt the pan from side to side until you get a thin layer of batter covering the base of the frying pan. Cook the pancake for about 1 minute, then flip it over (you can use a spatula for this) and cook until the underside is lightly flecked with gold. Continue with the rest of the batter, brushing the pan with melted butter when necessary.

French Toast

Makes 2 servings

1 large egg
2 tablespoons milk

2 thick slices of day-old white bread
1 tablespoon butter

Beat together the egg and milk and pour into a shallow dish. Cut the bread into triangles, or cut out shapes using cookie cutters. Dip the bread into the mixture and fry in the butter until golden. Serve with fruit or a fruit compote and dust with a little confectioners' or superfine sugar. (This is also good made with cinnamon raisin bread cut into fingers.)

Savory Breakfast Muffins

Cheese and tomato on toast makes a nutritious breakfast, and using split toasted English muffins makes a nice variation. You can vary the toppings depending on what you have on hand in the kitchen (see photograph).

Makes 1 or 2 servings

1 English muffin
Butter or margarine
1 tomato, sliced thinly
Salt and freshly ground black pepper
½ cup grated Cheddar cheese

Decoration
Thinly sliced ham
2 cherry tomatoes
2 slices of unpeeled cucumber
1 black olive

Split and toast the muffin. Spread with a little butter or margarine. Arrange some thinly sliced tomato on top, lightly season, and then cover with the grated cheese. Place under a preheated broiler until lightly golden. If you wish, you can then have some fun decorating the muffins to look like faces.

Apple and Carrot Breakfast Muffins

Here is a healthy and deliciously moist muffin that's bound to become a family favorite. These muffins are very easy to make and will keep well for up to 5 days. They are also great for lunch boxes or as a snack for any time of the day.

Makes 12 muffins

1 cup whole-wheat flour
¼ cup sugar
2 tablespoons nonfat dry milk
1½ teaspoons baking powder
½ teaspoon ground cinnamon
¼ teaspoon salt
¼ teaspoon ground ginger
½ cup vegetable oil

2 tablespoons honey
2 tablespoons maple syrup
2 eggs, lightly beaten
½ teaspoon pure vanilla extract
1 large apple, peeled and grated
½ cup grated carrot
½ cup raisins

Preheat the oven to 350°F. Combine the flour, sugar, nonfat dry milk, baking powder, cinnamon, salt, and ginger in a mixing bowl. In a separate bowl combine the oil, honey, maple syrup, eggs, and vanilla. Beat lightly with a wire whisk until blended. Add the grated apple, carrot, and raisins to the liquid mixture and stir well. Fold in the dry ingredients until just combined but don't overmix, or the muffins will become heavy.

Line a muffin tin with paper liners and fill the muffin cups until two-thirds full. Bake for 20 to 25 minutes.

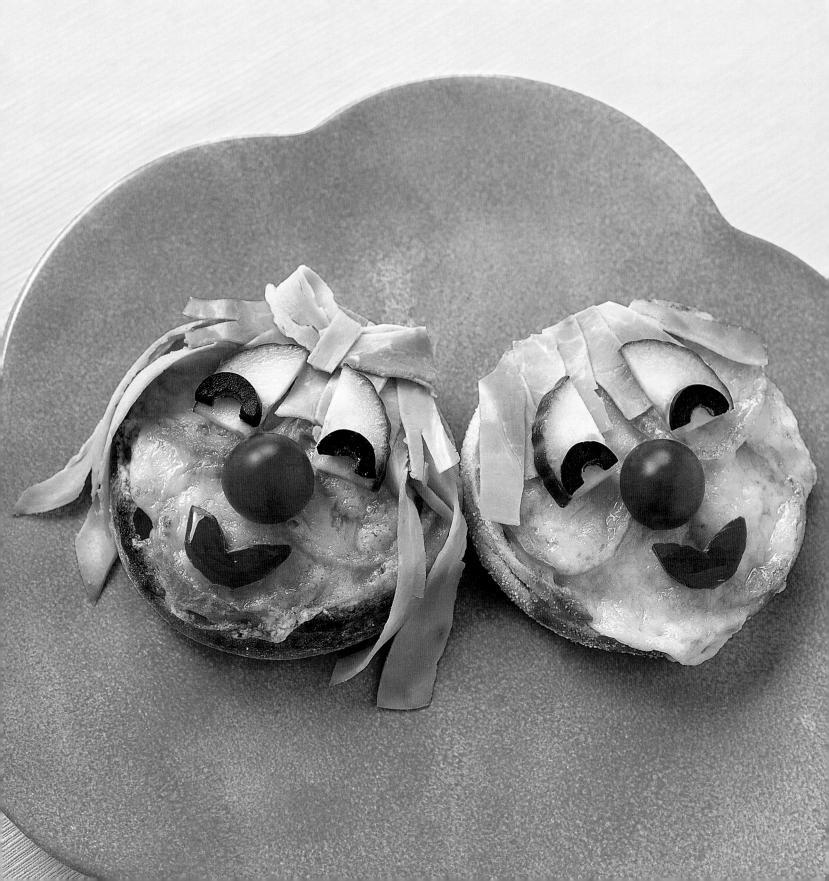

Fruity Homemade Muesli

So many of the breakfast cereals designed specifically for children are very high in sugar and low in nutrients. However, it's very easy to make your own delicious muesli using oats, fresh and dried fruits, and fresh fruit juices. There are now many delicious fresh fruit juices available in supermarkets, which can be used to soak and flavor the grains. This makes a nutritious alternative and you can add fresh fruit depending on the season (see photograph).

Makes 4 servings

2 cups rolled (not instant) oats
½ cup toasted wheat germ
¼ cup each dried peaches and apricots, finely chopped
2 tablespoons raisins
1½ cups apple and mango juice or apple juice

1 apple, peeled and grated
Fresh fruit, such as strawberries, raspberries, peaches

Soak the oats, toasted wheat germ, dried fruits, and raisins in the juice for at least 20 minutes or overnight. Stir in the grated apple and the fruit of your choice.

Delicious Homemade Granola

This makes a wonderfully nutritious breakfast. It is delicious on its own or with milk or yogurt and fresh fruit, and will keep for several weeks in an airtight container.

Makes 10 to 12 servings

One 12-ounce jar of honey
1 cup maple syrup
1 cup safflower or sunflower oil
2 teaspoons pure vanilla extract
4 cups rolled oats (organic are best)
½ cup sunflower seeds
½ cup pumpkin seeds

¼ cup bran
¼ cup wheat germ
¼ cup sesame seeds
1 cup slivered almonds
½ cup desiccated coconut
1 cup raisins
1 cup currants or dried cranberries

Preheat the oven to 300°F. In a saucepan, warm together the honey, maple syrup, safflower or sunflower oil, and vanilla. Combine the rolled oats, sunflower seeds, and pumpkin seeds and stir into the warm honey mixture. Spread out on a large baking sheet and bake for 10 minutes, stirring halfway through. Remove from the oven, mix in the bran, wheat germ, and sesame seeds and bake for 15 minutes, stirring occasionally. Spread the almonds and coconut on top and bake for another 15 minutes, stirring halfway through but still keeping the almonds on top. Finish off for about 4 minutes under a preheated broiler, watching to make sure that the mixture does not burn. Add the raisins and currants or cranberries. Allow to cool and transfer to an airtight container.

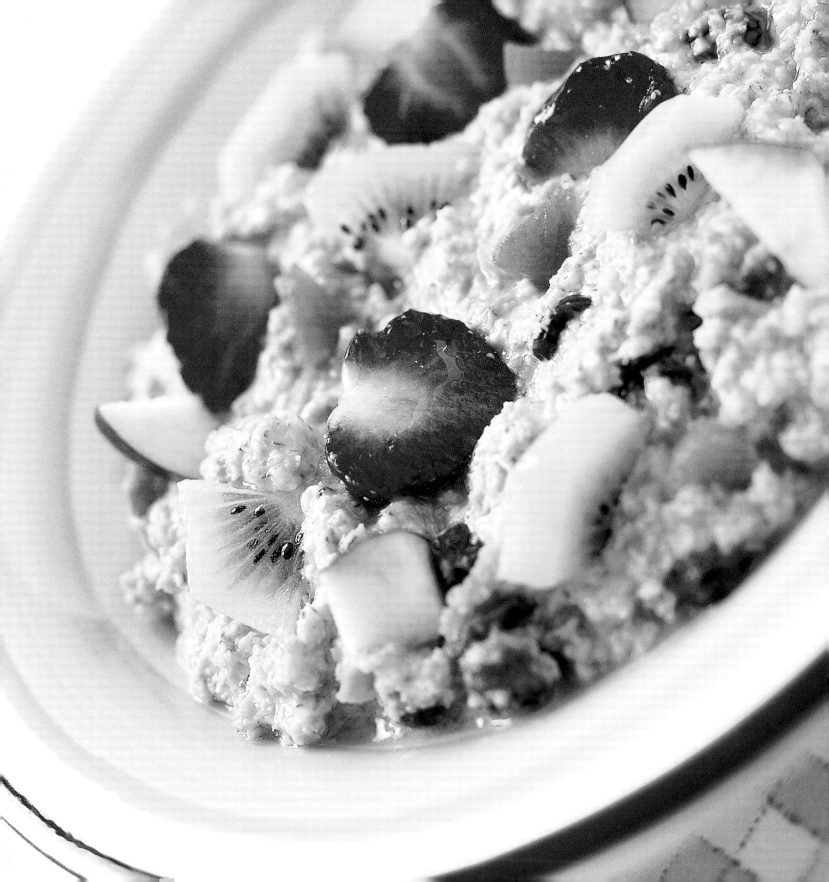

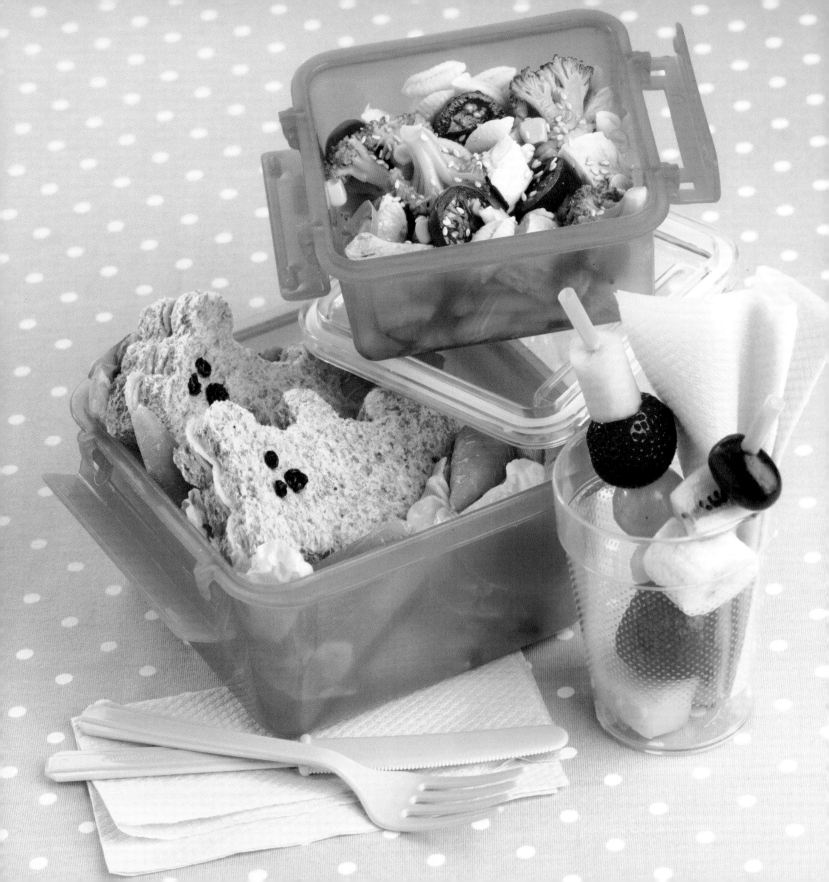

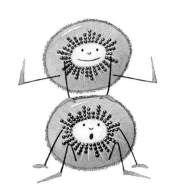

Soups, Snacks, and Lunch Boxes

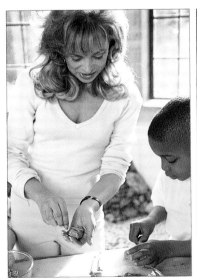
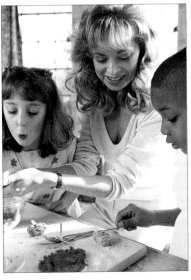
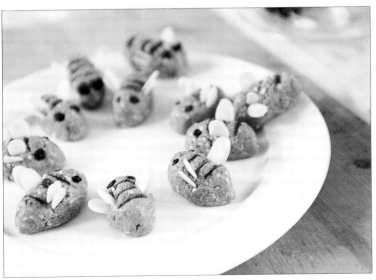

Soups, Snacks, and Lunch Boxes

PACKED LUNCHES

The nutritional quality of school meals varies hugely, and if you are unhappy with your child's school meals and are unable to effect any real changes to be sure that your child is getting a good balanced meal, a packed lunch may well be the sensible answer. Often fussy eaters will find nothing that they like to eat in the school dining room and may end up eating very little for lunch, with the consequence that they have no energy and lack concentration as the day wears on.

Warm conditions encourage the growth of bacteria, so it's important to keep lunch boxes cool. For the summer months buy some ice packs that can be frozen overnight and then popped into an insulated lunch box the next day to keep the food fresh. Alternatively, you can put a carton of juice in the freezer and transfer it to your child's lunch box in the morning; by lunchtime it will have defrosted but will have helped to keep your child's food fresh.

TOP TIPS

● Use lots of different breads such as pita bread, bagels, and ciabatta to make sandwiches. It's a good idea to have small plastic containers to put your sandwiches in so that they don't get squashed.

● Salads make a nice change from sandwiches: Try chicken caesar salad with cherry tomatoes and mini-balls of mozzarella, or turkey salad with pasta, whole kernel corn, cherry tomatoes, and scallions. Keep the salad dressing separate and let your child pour it over his salad himself so that it remains crisp.

● Avoid too many processed foods, as they tend to contain few nutrients and too much salt, sugar, additives, and saturated fat. If your child likes potato chips, but you don't want him to fill himself up by eating a whole bag,

put some in a small bag and tie the top. Try offering pretzels, toasted seeds, honey-roasted cashew nuts, or popcorn instead.

● Some foods such as pasta salads and sandwich fillings can be prepared the night before to save time in the morning, or use leftovers from a pasta dinner or homemade soup.

● As the colder weather sets in, it's a good idea to include something hot in a lunch box. A wide-mouthed mini thermos would be ideal for serving up a delicious cup of homemade or good-quality store-bought soup such as tomato soup, which is both warming and nutritious.

● Offer pure fruit juice, fruit smoothies, or water. Some juice drinks contain less than 10 percent juice and have 5 teaspoons of sugar added, so check the label before buying. Also many low-sugar drinks contain artificial sweeteners.

● Many cereal bars contain more than 40 percent sugar, and unlike the sugar in a bowl of cereal that gets washed away by the milk, this stuff sticks to your child's teeth.

● It is important to include fresh fruit in your child's lunch box—you can cut up wedges of mango, melon, papaya, and pineapple and pack them in a plastic container. Children tend to leave fruit that takes a lot of effort to eat, so when giving something such as tangerines, peel them first and wrap them in plastic wrap.

● Add a personal touch to your child's lunch; tuck in a note, stickers, or a joke or send a special treat labeled "Share with a friend." Pack fun napkins, decorate lunch bags with stickers, or draw a face on a banana with a Magic Marker.

Lunch Box Suggestions

✓ Crunchy raw vegetables with a tasty dip such as hummus or cream cheese and chives. Wrap sticks of carrot, cucumber, celery, and sweet pepper in damp paper towels to keep them fresh. Cherry tomatoes are also popular. You can also thread a variety of vegetables onto small wooden skewers and intersperse with cubes of cheese and maybe some rolled-up thinly sliced ham or turkey. Wrap in foil.

✓ Miniature cheeses from the supermarket—pick and mix selection.

✓ Yogurt, mini yogurt drinks, and flavored yogurts.

✓ A slice of pizza.

✓ Raisins and cashew nuts or honey-roasted cashew nuts.

✓ Dried fruit such as apricots. You can make fruit kebabs with different fruits, alternating fresh and dried.

✓ Include some home-baked cookies such as the Best-Ever Oatmeal Raisin Cookies on page 137. It's a good idea to get your child to help bake with you.

✓ Hard-boiled eggs.

✓ Chicken skewers—there are quite a variety in this book (see Teriyaki Chicken Skewers and Easy Yakitori Chicken on pages 55 and 68)—and they can be prepared the night before and refrigerated. These skewers are just as good cold as hot.

✓ Many supermarkets have individually wrapped snacks that are ideal to drop straight into your child's lunch box. Try such items as small cartons of fruit puree, mini yogurt drinks, twin cartons of cream cheese with miniature breadsticks, and miniature boxes of raisins.

✓ Vegetable chips: You can buy bags of crispy carrot, parsnip, sweet potato, and beet chips seasoned with sea salt.

✓ Rice cakes and other plain crackers.

✓ Cereal bars.

✓ A piece of fruit.

✓ Homemade or store-bought soup in a thermos.

Sandwich Fillings

Try some of these suggestions:

✓ Peanut butter and strawberry or raspberry jam

✓ Peanut butter, honey, and sliced banana

✓ Strawberry jam and plain cream cheese

✓ Cream cheese and cucumber

✓ Butter, shredded lettuce, and grated Cheddar cheese

✓ Peanut butter or chocolate spread and sliced banana

✓ Cheddar cheese with chutney, cucumber slices, or sliced pickles

✓ Shrimp salad mixed with a little ketchup

✓ Hard-boiled egg mashed with a little mayonnaise and sprinkled with chopped spinach, alfalfa sprouts, or some finely chopped celery

✓ Hummus, grated carrot, and sliced cucumber

✓ Cream cheese and chopped dried apricot

✓ Tuna salad with chopped celery

✓ Roast chicken or beef with salad in pita pockets

✓ Sliced turkey, lettuce, and Swiss cheese

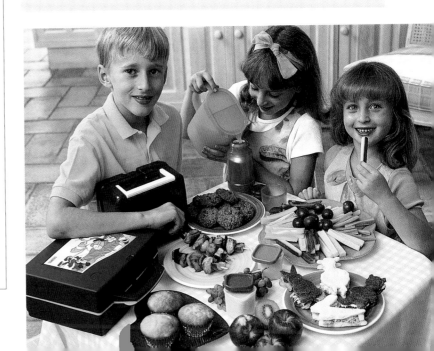

Lara's Lovely Onion Soup

My daughter Lara loves onion soup and this one is delicious, as I allow the onions to caramelize to bring out their flavor. You can mix ordinary onions with red onions if you like. It's great comfort food on a cold winter's night.

Makes 8 servings

2 tablespoons olive oil
4 tablespoons butter
1¼ pounds onions, thinly sliced
1 clove garlic, crushed
½ teaspoon sugar
4 cups beef stock

1 large potato, peeled and cubed
1 cup dry white wine
Salt and freshly ground black pepper
½ loaf French bread
¾ cup grated Swiss cheese

TIP

For winter, it's a good idea to include something hot in your child's lunch box, so invest in a small thermos that you can fill with soup. There are many delicious homemade soups to try, or perhaps heat up a small can of baked beans and use that to fill a thermos.

Heat the oil and butter in a large casserole. Add the onions, garlic, and sugar and cook over medium heat, stirring until the onions have browned. Reduce the heat to low, cover the onions with a sheet of nonstick baking paper, and leave the onions to cook slowly for 30 minutes.

Meanwhile, put 2 cups of the stock into a saucepan, add the potato, and cook for 10 to 12 minutes, or until the potato is soft. Blend the potato with some of the stock in a food processor or blender. This will help to thicken the soup.

Remove the nonstick baking paper and pour the thickened stock, the remaining beef stock, and the wine over the caramelized onions. Season, then stir with a wooden spoon, scraping the base of the pot to get the full flavor of the caramelized onions. Simmer gently, uncovered, for 30 minutes.

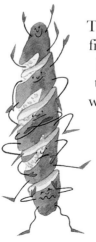

To make the cheesy French bread slices to float on top of the soup, first cut the loaf diagonally into ½-inch slices and toast lightly on both sides. Pour the soup into individual ovenproof bowls and top each one with a slice of bread. Sprinkle the bread liberally with the grated cheese. Place the bowls under the broiler until the cheese is melted and bubbling. Serve immediately.

Tasty and Healthy Vegetable Soup

A good homemade vegetable soup can be a great way to encourage reluctant vegetable eaters to eat more. This is one of my favorite combinations.

Makes 8 servings

1 tablespoon butter
1 medium onion, chopped
2½ cups (3 to 4 medium) chopped carrots
1 large potato, peeled and chopped
4 cups chicken or vegetable stock
1 cup chopped button mushrooms
1 celery stalk, chopped

1 clove garlic, crushed
½ teaspoon sugar
1½ teaspoons snipped fresh thyme
or ½ teaspoon dried thyme
Salt and freshly ground black pepper

Melt the butter in a large casserole or saucepan and sauté the onion until softened and lightly golden. Stir in the carrots and potato and cook, stirring, for 2 minutes. Pour over the stock and add the mushrooms, celery, garlic, sugar, and thyme. Bring to a boil, then reduce the heat and simmer, covered, for about 50 minutes. Puree in a blender and season to taste.

Nourishing Lentil Soup

Lentils are not generally very popular with children, but here's a very tasty way to enjoy them. This nutritious soup has proved very popular with my young team of tasters, who never hesitate to give something the thumbs down if it doesn't appeal.

Makes 8 servings

1 tablespoon butter
1 medium onion, chopped
1 leek, white part only, finely sliced
1 clove garlic, crushed
1½ cups (about 2 medium) chopped carrots
¼ cup finely sliced celery

1 cup red lentils
1 medium potato, peeled and diced
2 tablespoons chopped fresh parsley
6 cups vegetable or chicken stock
Salt and freshly ground black pepper

Melt the butter in a large saucepan and sauté the onion, leek, garlic, carrots, and celery for about 10 minutes or until softened. Add the lentils, diced potato, and parsley and pour the stock into the mixture. Stir and bring to a boil. Season with a little salt and freshly ground black pepper, cover, and simmer gently for about 45 minutes. Puree in a blender to a thick, smooth consistency.

Thai-Style Chicken Soup

Thai-style food tends to be very popular with children, and this quick, easy-to-prepare soup is almost a meal in itself. Add more chile if you want to spice it up a little.

Makes 4 servings

1 tablespoon light olive oil
1 medium onion, chopped
1 clove garlic, crushed (bash the garlic
to make it easy to peel)
½ red chile, finely chopped (approximately
1 tablespoon)

1 boneless, skinless chicken breast, cut into thin strips
1 cup broccoli florets
2 cups chicken stock
1 cup coconut milk
Salt and freshly ground black pepper
¾ cup cooked rice (¼ cup raw)

Heat the oil in a pan and sauté the onion, garlic, and chile for 2 minutes. Add the strips of chicken and sauté for 2 more minutes. Add the broccoli and chicken stock, bring to a boil, and simmer for 4 minutes. Stir in the coconut milk and simmer for 2 minutes. Season to taste and stir in the cooked rice.

Mummy's Minestrone

Minestrone is a family favorite in our house. Sometimes, I leave out the baked beans and soup pasta and instead add a can of cartoon character pasta in tomato sauce, which seems to add to its child appeal.

Makes 8 servings

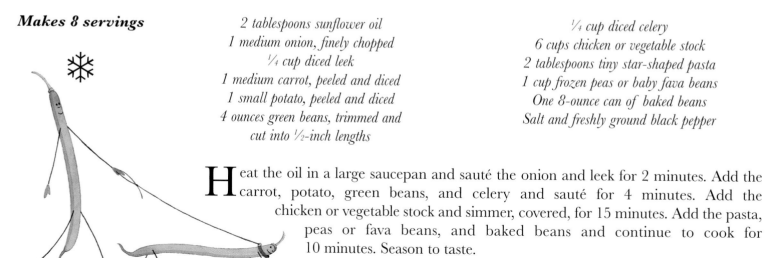

2 tablespoons sunflower oil
1 medium onion, finely chopped
¼ cup diced leek
1 medium carrot, peeled and diced
1 small potato, peeled and diced
4 ounces green beans, trimmed and
cut into ½-inch lengths

¼ cup diced celery
6 cups chicken or vegetable stock
2 tablespoons tiny star-shaped pasta
1 cup frozen peas or baby fava beans
One 8-ounce can of baked beans
Salt and freshly ground black pepper

Heat the oil in a large saucepan and sauté the onion and leek for 2 minutes. Add the carrot, potato, green beans, and celery and sauté for 4 minutes. Add the chicken or vegetable stock and simmer, covered, for 15 minutes. Add the pasta, peas or fava beans, and baked beans and continue to cook for 10 minutes. Season to taste.

Mediterranean Tomato Soup

This tomato soup has a wonderful flavor and it's a great recipe to encourage children to eat more vegetables. Tomatoes are particularly rich in vitamin C and lycopene (the red pigment), which has been found to help protect against certain forms of cancer, in particular prostate cancer, so it's especially advisable for men to include tomatoes in their diet several times a week. Lycopene is released when tomatoes are cooked and better absorbed with a little oil.

Makes 6 servings

2 tablespoons olive oil
2 tablespoons butter
2 medium onions, diced
2 medium carrots, peeled and diced
2 celery stalks, diced
1 clove garlic, crushed
1½ tablespoons roughly chopped fresh basil

1½ tablespoons roughly chopped fresh tarragon
1 bay leaf
1 pound ripe plum tomatoes, peeled, quartered, and seeded
One 14-ounce can of chopped tomatoes
1 tablespoon tomato paste
2 cups chicken stock
Salt and freshly ground black pepper

Heat the olive oil and butter in a large saucepan and sauté the onions, carrots, and celery for 2 to 3 minutes. Add the garlic, herbs, and bay leaf and cook for 7 to 8 minutes. Add the fresh and canned tomatoes and cook over low heat for about 15 minutes. Stir in the tomato paste and gradually add the stock. Cook over medium heat for 15 minutes. Remove the bay leaf and blend in a food processor or blender. Season to taste.

Tuna Melt

Try this nutritious, tasty, quick, and easy snack. If you wish you can use low-fat sour cream and Cheddar cheese.

Makes 2 servings

One 6-ounce can of tuna in water
2 tablespoons ketchup
2 tablespoons crème fraîche or plain yogurt

1 to 2 finely sliced scallions (optional)
2 English muffins
2 tablespoons grated Cheddar cheese

Drain the water from the tuna and flake into small pieces. Mix together with the ketchup, crème fraîche or yogurt, and scallions, if using.

Split the muffins and toast them. Spread with the tuna mixture and sprinkle with the grated Cheddar. Place the muffins under a preheated broiler and broil until the cheese is golden and bubbling.

Cucumber Crocodile

This looks amazing, it's great for parties, and it also makes a fabulous prop for your own children's healthy snacks. I like to use a variety of cheeses, but cubes of ham or chicken also work well in place of the cheese (see photograph).

Makes 4 to 6 servings

1 carrot
1¼ unpeeled cucumbers
Mixture of cheeses

Fresh pineapple, cut into chunks, or
1 small can of pineapple chunks
2 cherry tomatoes

Cut a long strip from the carrot using a vegetable peeler. Cut this into a strip about ½ inch wide and cut along one side to form a serrated edge. These are the crocodile's teeth. Cut a wedge from the end of the cucumber to make its mouth. Cut the ¼ cucumber into two 1-inch-wide slices, cut these in half, and then shape into feet with a triangular shape cut out of them. Attach these to the whole cucumber using toothpicks cut in half. Chop the cheese and pineapple into cubes. Thread a cheese and pineapple cube onto each toothpick and spear the end into the cucumber. Cut a toothpick in half and use the two halves to attach the cherry tomatoes to form the crocodile's eyes.

Bagel Fillers

Bagels are popular for a tasty snack or for your child's lunch box. They are great with so many different fillings. You can also toast the bagels.

Good Bagel Fillings
Cream cheese, smoked salmon, lemon juice,
and black pepper
Pastrami and gherkins
Small shrimp mixed with mayonnaise, a little
ketchup, and Worcestershire sauce, and
sprinkled with paprika
Chopped cooked chicken with chopped hard-boiled
egg, corn, mayonnaise, and
chopped sun-dried tomatoes

Crispy cooked slices of bacon
with a few crisp lettuce leaves, sliced tomato,
and a little mayonnaise
Sliced turkey, Swiss cheese, tomato, lettuce,
and salad dressing
Flaked tuna with corn, scallion,
and mayonnaise
Sliced ham and Swiss cheese
Egg salad and spinach or lettuce

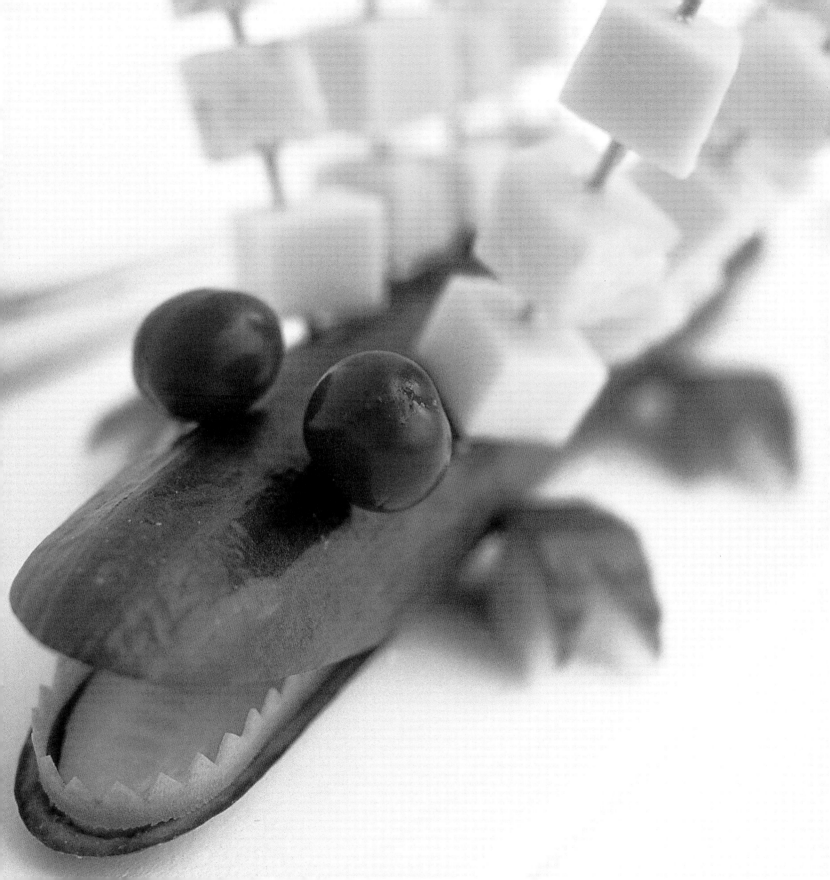

Turkey Pasta Salad

A quick and easy salad that is very nutritious. Great for lunch boxes or a light snack.
This has a really nice dressing that children love!

Makes 2 or 3 servings

¼ cup pasta shapes
½ cup broccoli florets
3½ ounces cooked turkey or chicken breast, chopped
¾ cup canned or frozen corn
2 tomatoes, peeled, seeded, and chopped,
or 6 cherry tomatoes, halved
2 scallions, thinly sliced
1 tablespoon toasted sesame seeds

Dressing
3 tablespoons light olive oil
1 tablespoon honey
1 tablespoon soy sauce
1 tablespoon lemon juice

Cook the pasta in lightly salted boiling water according to the instructions on the package. Steam the broccoli florets for 5 minutes. Meanwhile, whisk together all the ingredients for the dressing.

Put the turkey or chicken, corn, tomatoes, and scallions into a bowl together with the drained pasta and the broccoli and toss with the dressing.

> **Tortilla wraps make a nice change from ordinary sandwiches. Try fillings such as:**
> - Cooked chicken, salsa, and sour cream
> - Hummus and grated carrot
> - Sliced turkey with shredded lettuce, grated Cheddar cheese, and salad dressing

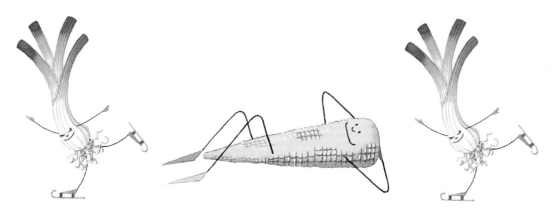

Mini English Muffin Pizzas

These mini-pizzas are delicious. I have used a zucchini and cherry tomato topping, but you can choose any topping, perhaps adding some diced ham on top of the tomato sauce before covering with grated cheese. Otherwise, just make a simple cheese and tomato pizza without any extra toppings. You can double the quantity of tomato sauce and keep it in the refrigerator ready for when you want to make pizzas. You can also make these using chilled pizza dough bought in the supermarket, which you simply roll out and cut into circles. Follow the instructions on the package.

Makes 4 mini pizzas

1 tablespoon olive oil
½ small onion, finely chopped
1 small clove garlic, crushed
½ cup tomato puree
1½ teaspoons tomato paste
Pinch of sugar
Salt and freshly ground black pepper
1 tablespoon torn fresh basil (optional)
2 English muffins, halved
¾ cup grated Cheddar or mozzarella cheese,
or a mixture of both

Toppings
Sliced salami
Pepperoni
Diced ham and pineapple
Corn
Sweet pepper
Mushrooms
Sliced pitted olives
Cherry tomatoes
Basil

Heat the olive oil in a small saucepan and sauté the onion and garlic for 3 to 4 minutes. Add the tomato puree together with the tomato paste, sugar, and a little seasoning and cook for approximately 2 minutes or until the mixture is thick enough to spread. Remove from the heat and stir in the torn basil leaves, if using.

Toast the split muffins and divide the tomato sauce between them. Choose your favorite topping and then cover with the grated cheese. Place under a preheated broiler until golden and bubbling.

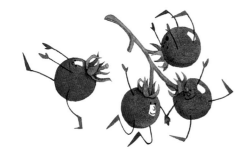
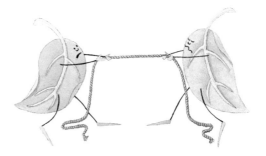
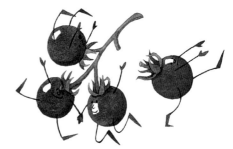

Buzzy Bees

These tasty bees are great fun for parties and they are just the right size for little children. They are packed full of nutritious ingredients, and older children will also enjoy making these themselves because they are quick and easy to make and need no cooking. You may want to double the quantity next time around, since these bees will keep your children buzzing around for more.

Makes 10 bees

¼ cup smooth peanut butter
1 tablespoon honey
2 tablespoons nonfat dry milk
1 tablespoon sesame seeds
1 shredded wheat biscuit, crushed

Decoration

1 tablespoon cocoa powder
Sliced almonds, or rice paper
cut into the shape of wings
10 currants

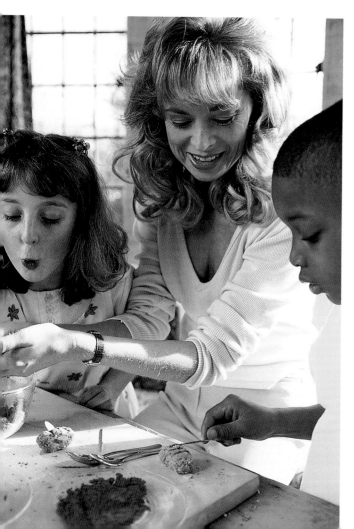

Mix together the peanut butter and honey, then blend in the remaining ingredients. Form heaping teaspoons of the mixture into oval shapes to look like bees. To decorate, dip a toothpick into the cocoa powder and press gently onto the bees' bodies to form stripes. Press sliced almonds or rice paper wings into the sides of the bees. Cut the currants in half, roll between your finger and thumb to form tiny balls, and arrange them on the bees to look like eyes. The bees can be stored in the refrigerator for several days.

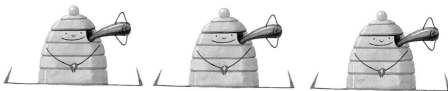

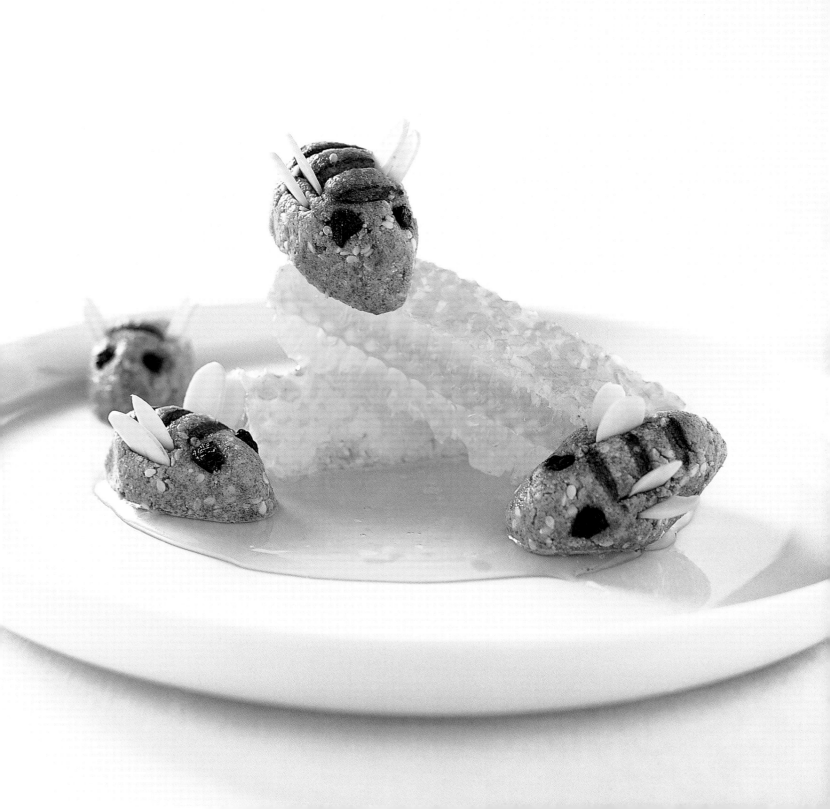

Salad Bar with Soy Sauce Dressing

Salads and a baked potato can easily become a main meal with the addition of ingredients such as grated cheese, chopped egg, or chopped chicken. Combined with some delicious freshly baked breads, which can now be bought in the supermarket, fresh fruit, and ice cream, this makes an easy and popular meal for the whole family. Sometimes when I have a group of children over for lunch in the summer, I lay out a salad bar with bowls of different ingredients and a choice of dressings so that everyone can help themselves. The Dressing for Dinner sauce (page 29) is my favorite and is particularly popular with my children. Here are some ideas for your salad bar.

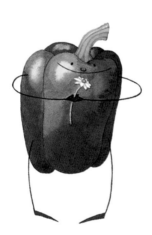

A variety of different lettuces
Cherry tomatoes
Cucumber
Grated carrot
Sweet peppers
Tiny florets of broccoli or cauliflower
Cooked green beans
Cooked corn
Hard-boiled egg
Toasted sunflower seeds
Avocado tossed in lemon juice
Pine nuts
Tuna fish
Grated cheese or chopped blue cheese
Cooked pasta
Chopped chicken or turkey

Soy Sauce Dressing
1 tablespoon balsamic or wine vinegar
Generous pinch of ground mustard
Pinch of superfine sugar
1 tablespoon soy sauce
Freshly ground black pepper
¼ cup light olive oil

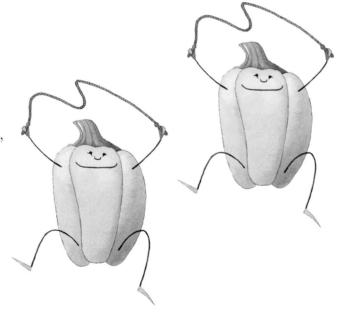

To make the dressing, mix together the first five ingredients, then whisk in the olive oil.

Salad Bar with Soy Sauce Dressing is shown on pages 30–31.

Japanese Salad Dressing

This dressing is pure magic, and I can't make enough of it to please my children. It is based on the salad dressing served at a chain of popular restaurants called Benihana. I use it to dress a mixed salad of crisp mixed lettuce, tomatoes, grated carrot, cucumber, and sometimes thinly sliced radish. Once you've tried this recipe you will probably want to increase the quantities and keep a bottleful in your refrigerator.

Makes 6 servings

1 tablespoon soy sauce
¼ cup light sour cream
½ teaspoon minced or finely chopped fresh gingerroot

2 teaspoons superfine sugar
2 tablespoons rice wine vinegar

Combine the soy sauce, sour cream, gingerroot, sugar, and vinegar with an electric handheld blender and blend until smooth.

Dressing for Dinner

The secret of getting your child to enjoy eating salad is to make a seductive salad dressing. My children are all hooked on this dressing and now prefer to come home to a plate of delicious salad vegetables rather than to a bag of potato chips and a chocolate cookie.

Makes 5 servings

¼ cup finely chopped onion
¼ cup vegetable oil
2 tablespoons rice wine vinegar
2 tablespoons water
1½ teaspoons chopped fresh gingerroot
1 tablespoon chopped celery

1 tablespoon soy sauce
1½ teaspoons tomato paste
1½ teaspoons sugar
1 teaspoon lemon juice
Salt and freshly ground black pepper

Combine all the ingredients, except for the salt and pepper, in a blender or food processor and process until smooth. Season to taste.

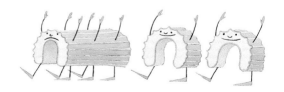

TIP
Dressing for Dinner is also good mixed with a pasta salad of cooked pasta shapes, steamed cauliflower, green beans, corn, diced tomato, and some diced cooked chicken. It also makes an excellent salad for your child's lunch box.

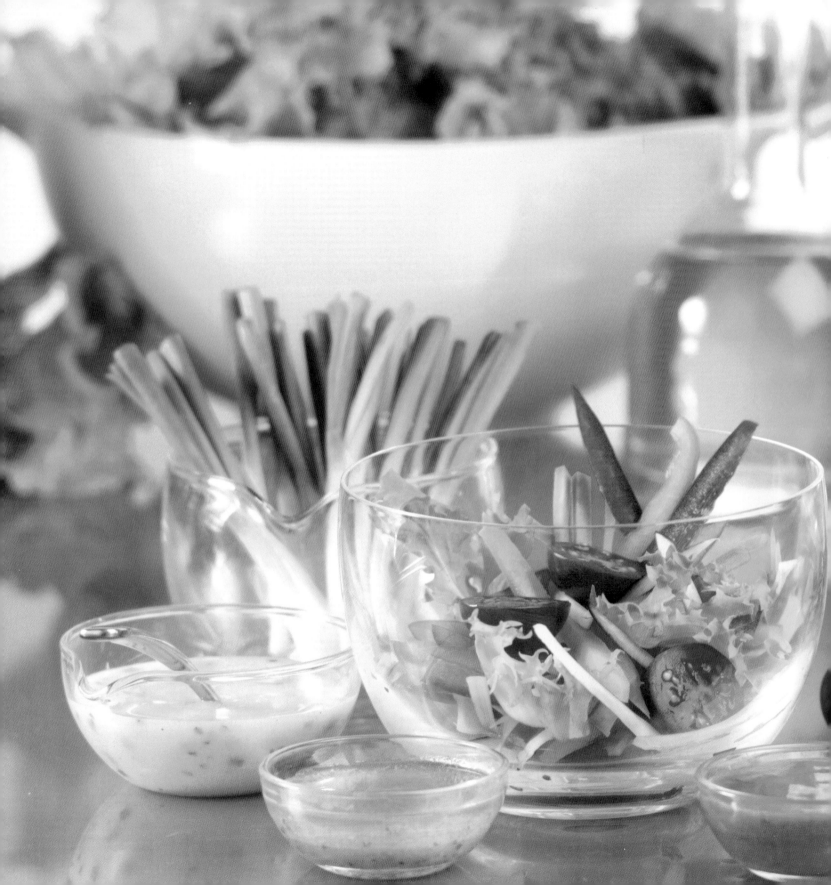

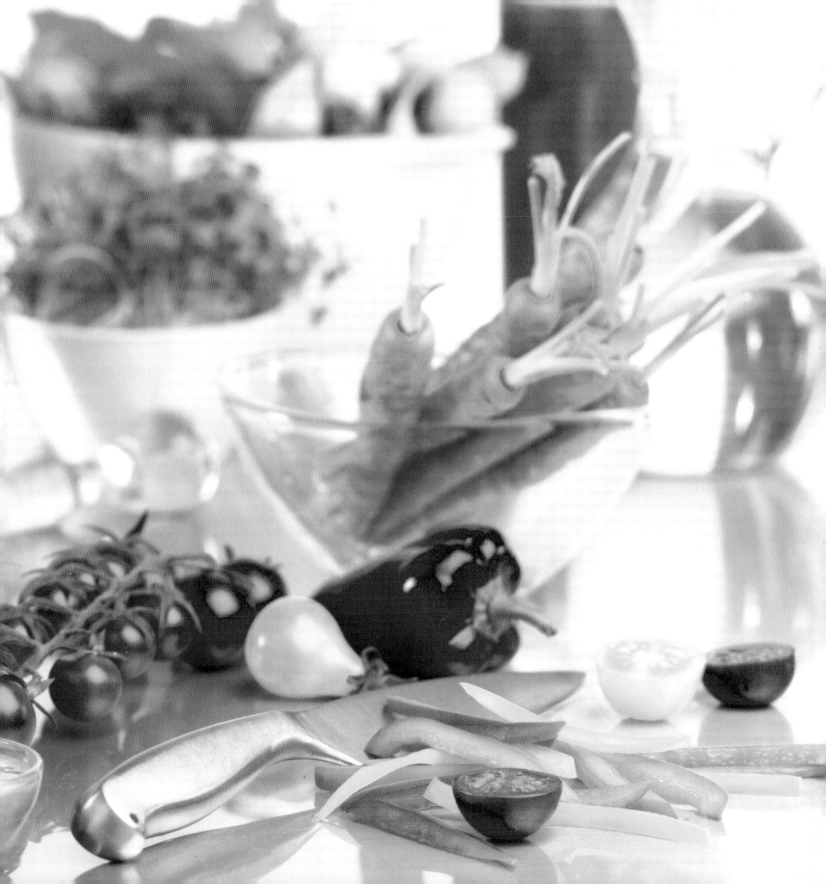

Bagel Snake

This is a fun way of arranging sandwiches, and I find that bagels are popular with both children and their moms and dads. You can make the snake as long as you like, depending on how many bagels you use, and you can use a variety of toppings. I have chosen tuna and egg toppings, which are both nutritious, but, of course, there is an infinite variety of ingredients that you can choose, such as cream cheese and cucumber.

Makes 2 servings

2 bagels

Tuna Salad Topping
One 6-ounce can of tuna in olive oil (drained)
2 tablespoons ketchup
2 tablespoons crème fraîche or plain yogurt
2 scallions, finely sliced

Egg Salad Topping
2 to 3 hard-boiled eggs
3 tablespoons mayonnaise
1 tablespoon snipped fresh chives
Salt and freshly ground black pepper

Decoration
Cherry tomatoes, halved
Chives
1 stuffed olive, sliced
Strip of sweet red pepper

Slice the bagels in half and then cut each half down the center to form a semicircle. Cut out the head of the snake from one of the pieces of bagel and the tail from another. Mix the ingredients for the tuna salad topping and mix the ingredients for the egg salad topping. Spread half the bagels with tuna and half with egg.

Decorate the tuna salad topping with halved cherry tomatoes and the egg salad topping with strips of chive arranged in a crisscross pattern. Arrange the bagels to form the body of a snake. Then attach the head to the snake's body and arrange two slices of stuffed olive to form the eyes and cut out a forked tongue from the strip of red pepper.

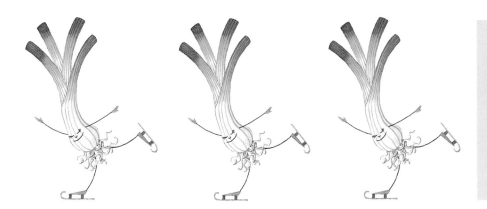

NOVELTY-SHAPED SANDWICHES
Use cookie cutters to cut sandwiches into shapes such as animals or gingerbread people. This really is an easy way of transforming a simple sandwich into something special for your child. It can also be a particularly good way of tempting the reluctant sandwich eater, especially since the crusts are removed.

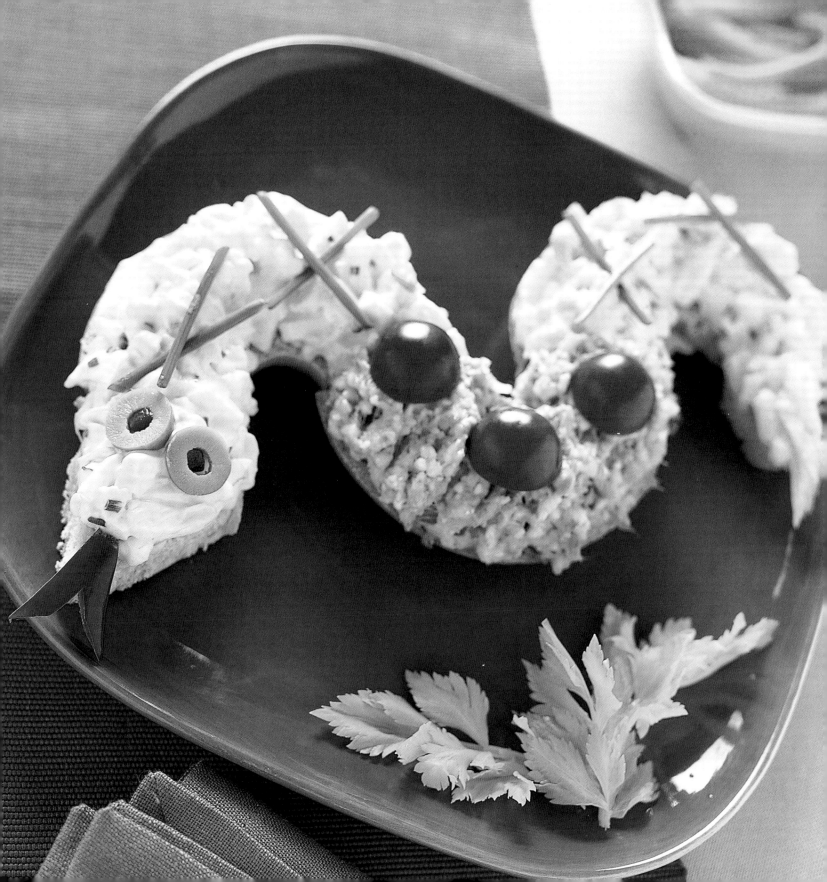

Cheesy Pretzels

These make good snacks, and children will have great fun twisting them into different shapes.

Makes 12 to 14 pretzels

2 cups all-purpose flour
¼ cup grated Cheddar cheese
2 tablespoons butter, diced
2 teaspoons baking powder
1 teaspoon sugar
½ teaspoon salt
⅓ cup milk
1 egg, lightly beaten

Toppings
Coarse sea salt
Sesame seeds
Extra grated cheese

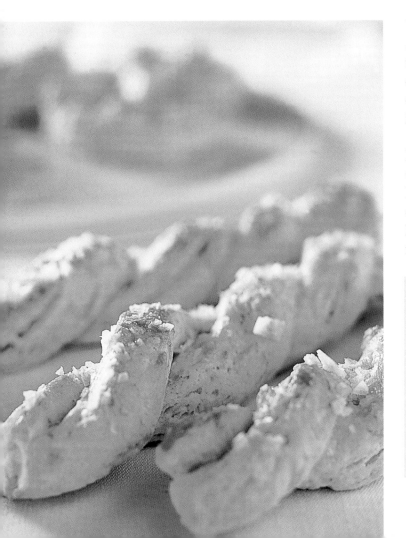

Preheat the oven to 400°F. Put the flour, cheese, butter, baking powder, sugar, and salt in a mixing bowl and mix together with your fingers. Gradually add the milk to form a ball of dough. Sprinkle a clean surface with some flour and roll the dough around 3 to 4 times. Knead the dough by folding, pressing, and turning and repeat this about 10 times.

Roll out the dough to a rectangle measuring about 10 x 7 inches. Cut the dough lengthwise into strips, each about ½ inch wide. Pinch the edges and twist each strip into a pretzel shape. Place on a greased baking sheet, brush with the beaten egg, and sprinkle with salt and sesame seeds or some extra grated cheese. Bake for 10 to 12 minutes or until golden.

A BALANCED LUNCH BOX

A packed lunch should contain:

✓ A high carbohydrate food, such as sandwiches or pasta salad
✓ Some protein, such as cheese, chicken drumstick, or tuna
✓ Fresh fruit
✓ Something sweet and nutritious, such as a muffin or cereal bar
✓ A drink, such as pure fruit juice, milk, or yogurt

Try to choose plenty of fresh foods and not too many highly refined foods.

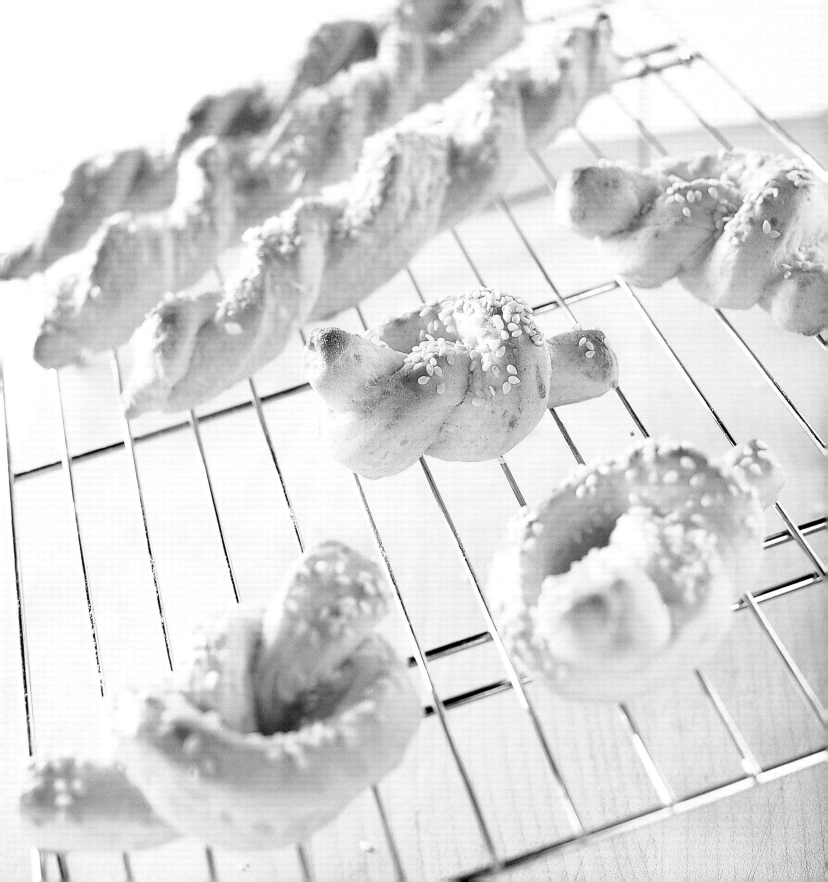

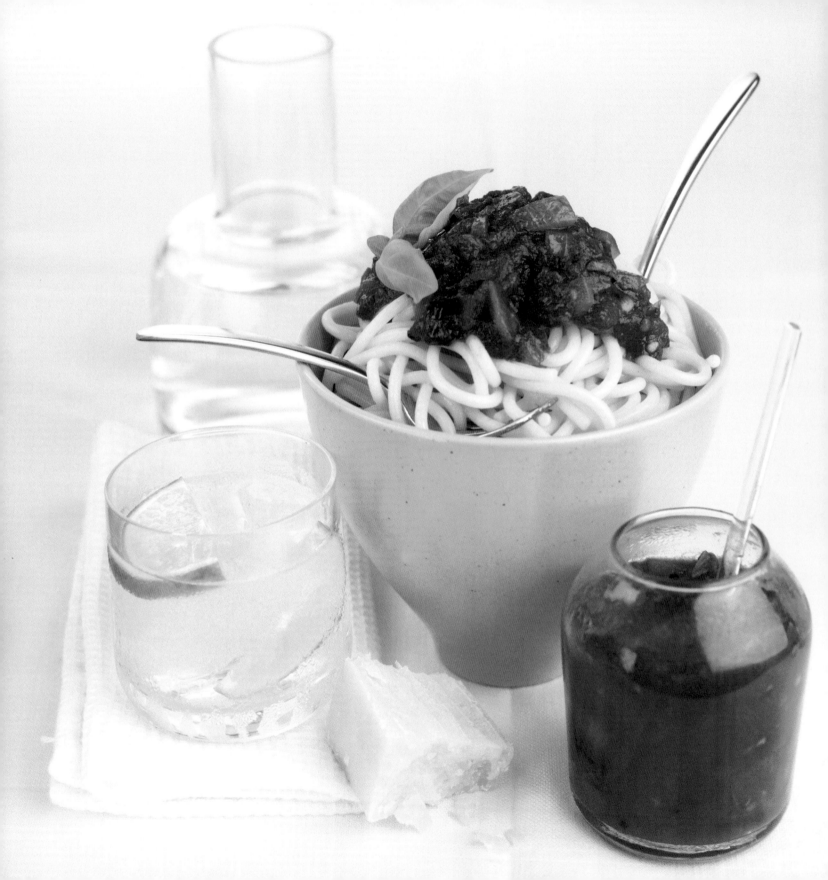

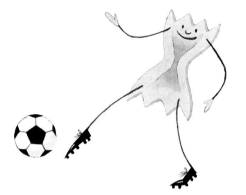

Pasta

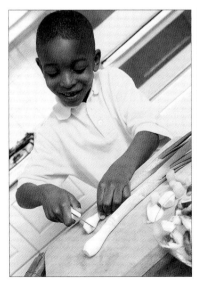

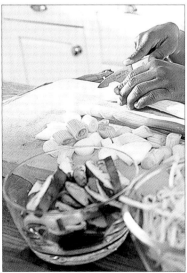

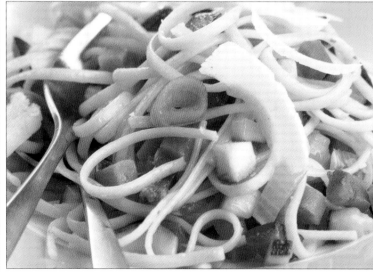

Annabel's 15-Minute Tomato Sauce

There are now lots of wonderful ingredients available in most supermarkets such as pesto and fresh basil, which can transform an ordinary tomato sauce into something very special. Vary the sauce by adding some sliced sautéed mushrooms.

Makes 4 servings

1 small onion, finely chopped
1 clove garlic, crushed
¼ to ½ teaspoon finely chopped red chile (optional)
2 tablespoons olive oil
Two 14-ounce cans of chopped tomatoes
2 tablespoons red pesto

1 teaspoon balsamic vinegar
1 teaspoon sugar
Salt and freshly ground black pepper
1 tablespoon torn fresh basil
¼ cup grated Parmesan cheese
8 ounces spaghettini

Sauté the onion, garlic, and chile, if using, in the olive oil for about 5 minutes. Drain the juice from one of the cans of tomatoes and stir in the drained tomatoes and the second can of tomatoes and juice. Add all the other ingredients except the basil and Parmesan cheese, stir, and let simmer for 10 minutes. Stir in the basil and Parmesan cheese and let simmer until the cheese is melted.

Meanwhile, cook the spaghettini according to the instructions on the package. Drain and serve topped with the sauce.

Lara's Lasagne

This is one of my daughter Lara's favorite dishes, and in winter it makes a good family meal and freezes well. Lasagne seems to be one of those dishes that are popular with most children. It provides a good source of iron and calcium.

Makes 6 servings

1 tablespoon olive oil
1 medium onion, chopped
1 clove garlic, crushed
½ sweet red pepper, cored, seeded, and chopped
1 pound lean ground beef
½ teaspoon mixed dried herbs
One 14-ounce can of chopped tomatoes, drained
One 10¾-ounce can of condensed cream of tomato soup
Salt and freshly ground black pepper

Cheese Sauce
4 tablespoons butter
¼ cup all-purpose flour
2 cups milk
Generous pinch of ground nutmeg
Salt and freshly ground black pepper
½ cup grated Swiss cheese

9 sheets of fresh or no-boil lasagne
¼ cup grated Parmesan cheese

Preheat the oven to 375°F. Heat the oil in a large saucepan and sauté the onion, garlic, and red pepper until softened. Add the beef and herbs and sauté until the beef has changed color. Add the tomatoes and soup and cook over medium heat for 15 to 20 minutes. Season to taste.

Meanwhile, to prepare the cheese sauce, melt the butter, stir in the flour, and cook for 1 minute. Gradually whisk in the milk, bring to a boil, and whisk until thickened and smooth. Season with the nutmeg and a little salt and pepper. Remove from the heat and stir in the grated Swiss cheese until melted.

To assemble the lasagne, spoon a little of the meat sauce onto the base of an ovenproof dish measuring 11 x 7 x 2 inches. Cover with 3 sheets of the lasagne. Divide the remaining meat sauce in half and cover the lasagne with half of the sauce. Spoon over a little of the cheese sauce.

Cover with 3 more sheets of the lasagne and cover with the remaining meat sauce. Again spoon over a little of the cheese sauce, but make sure that enough remains to completely cover the top layer of lasagne. Arrange the remaining 3 sheets of lasagne on top and then spread over the remaining cheese sauce so that the lasagne is completely covered. Sprinkle on the Parmesan cheese and bake in the oven for 25 to 30 minutes.

Spaghetti with Plum Tomatoes and Basil

A really good homemade tomato sauce is always popular and can be served with any type of pasta and some freshly grated Parmesan cheese. You can add a couple of tablespoons of chopped sun-dried tomatoes together with the fresh tomatoes if you want to bring out the flavor. The sauce can be frozen separately (see photograph, page 36).

Makes 4 servings

2 tablespoons olive oil
1 medium onion, chopped
1 clove garlic, crushed
4 ripe plum tomatoes, peeled, seeded, and chopped
One 14-ounce can of chopped tomatoes

½ teaspoon balsamic vinegar
½ teaspoon brown sugar
Handful of basil leaves, torn into pieces
Salt and freshly ground black pepper
8 ounces spaghetti

Heat the oil in a saucepan and sauté the onion and garlic for 5 to 6 minutes, until softened but not colored. Add the remaining ingredients (except the spaghetti), cover, and cook over medium heat for about 20 minutes.

Meanwhile, bring a large pot of lightly salted water to a boil. Add the spaghetti and cook according to the instructions on the package. Drain and serve topped with the sauce.

Orient Express

Stir-fries are easy and quick to prepare, as everything is cooked in the same pan, and they make a great family meal. As a shortcut you can buy a pre-cut selection of stir-fry vegetables from your local supermarket. This can also be made with 10 ounces of beef cut into strips instead of the chicken. If you have some large carrots, it's fun to cut the carrot slices into stars using mini cookie cutters. Serve with rice or noodles. For extra appeal, how about using some "child friendly" chopsticks made from brightly colored plastic, which are joined at the top.

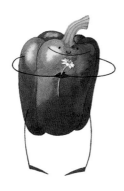

Makes 6 servings

Marinade
1 tablespoon soy sauce
1 tablespoon sake or sherry
1 teaspoon sesame oil
1 teaspoon cornstarch

*2 boneless, skinless chicken breasts,
cut into strips*
8 ounces pasta twirls
3 tablespoons vegetable oil
2 eggs, lightly beaten
1 medium onion, finely sliced

1 clove garlic, chopped (optional)
1 cup small broccoli florets
8 canned whole baby corn, cut in half
½ sweet red pepper, cut into strips
*1 medium carrot, peeled and cut into stars
or strips*
½ cup sliced button mushrooms
2 tablespoons finely sliced scallions
1½ to 2 tablespoons oyster sauce
*1 chicken stock cube dissolved in 6 tablespoons
boiling water*
Freshly ground black pepper

Mix together the ingredients for the marinade and marinate the chicken for about 30 minutes. Cook the pasta in a large pot of lightly salted boiling water according to the package instructions. Drain and set aside.

In a frying pan, heat 1½ teaspoons of the oil and fry the eggs until set. Cut into strips and set aside. Then heat 1 tablespoon of the oil in a wok or large frying pan and stir-fry half the onion and garlic, if using, for 2 to 3 minutes. Add the chicken and marinade and stir-fry until the chicken is cooked through. Remove the chicken and onion and set aside.

Heat the remaining 1½ tablespoons oil in the wok or frying pan and stir-fry the rest of the onion and garlic for 2 to 3 minutes. Add the broccoli, baby corn, red pepper, and carrot and stir-fry for about 5 minutes. Sprinkle over a little water while stir-frying the vegetables. Add the mushrooms and scallions and cook for 2 to 3 minutes.

Return the chicken to the wok, add the oyster sauce and stock, and continue to cook for 2 to 3 minutes or until the vegetables are tender and the chicken is cooked through. Add the pasta and stir to combine. Season with freshly ground black pepper.

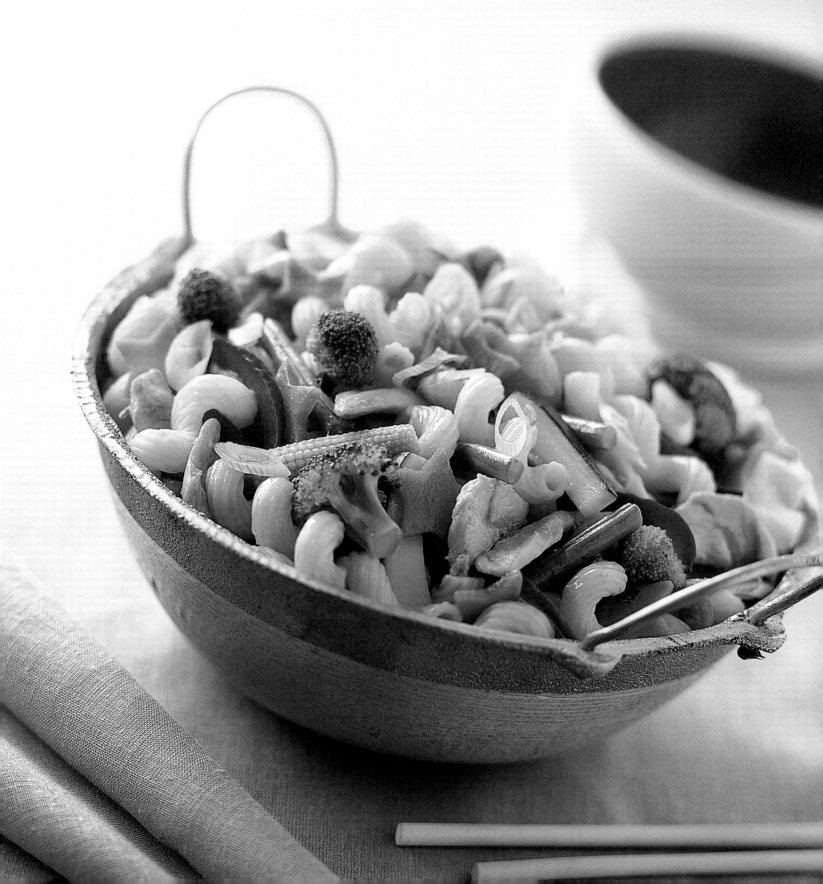

Easy Bolognese Sauce

This is a very quick and easy way to make a bolognese sauce using a can of tomato soup as one of the ingredients. Since red meat provides the best source of iron, it's good to find some family favorites that include it, and this pasta sauce is particularly appealing to children.

Makes 4 adult or 8 child servings

1 large onion, chopped
1 clove garlic, crushed
1 tablespoon vegetable oil
1 pound lean ground beef
½ teaspoon mixed dried herbs

1 cup sliced button mushrooms
One 14-ounce can of chopped tomatoes
One 10¾-ounce can of condensed cream of tomato soup
Salt and freshly ground black pepper
1 pound spaghetti

Sauté the onion and garlic in the oil for 2 to 3 minutes. Add the beef and herbs and sauté until the beef has changed color. Add the sliced mushrooms and sauté for 2 minutes. Add the tomatoes and soup and cook over medium heat for about 15 minutes. Season to taste. Meanwhile, cook the spaghetti in a large pot of lightly salted boiling water according to the instructions on the package. Drain the cooked pasta and mix with the bolognese sauce and serve.

Three-Cheese Macaroni

Pasta provides a good source of complex carbohydrates, so this macaroni will boost your child's energy level as well as providing a good source of protein and calcium. For a meaty version, add some chopped bacon or ham.

Makes 4 servings

8 ounces elbow macaroni or other pasta shape
2 tablespoons butter
2 tablespoons all-purpose flour
2 cups milk
Generous pinch of ground nutmeg

½ cup grated Cheddar cheese
½ cup grated Swiss cheese
Salt and freshly ground black pepper
3 tablespoons grated Parmesan cheese

Cook the elbow macaroni or other pasta shape in a large pot of lightly salted boiling water according to the instructions on the package. Drain thoroughly. Melt the butter in a pan, stir in the flour, and cook, stirring, for 1 minute. Gradually whisk in the milk and nutmeg, bring to a boil, and then simmer for a few minutes to make a smooth sauce.

Remove from the heat and stir in the Cheddar and Swiss until melted. Season to taste. Add the drained pasta and stir to combine. Transfer to an ovenproof dish, sprinkle with the Parmesan, and place under a preheated broiler until the top is golden.

Lasagne with Spinach, Cheese, and Tomato

This is my favorite vegetarian lasagne. If you can find sheets of fresh lasagne, I think they taste better than dried, and some supermarkets stock them in the refrigerated section. If using the dried lasagne, you may need to cook this for 5 minutes longer and make sure that the lasagne is completely covered with sauce or it will dry out.

Makes 4 servings

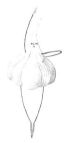

Tomato Sauce
1 medium onion, chopped
1 clove garlic, crushed
1 tablespoon olive oil
2 tablespoons tomato paste
Two 14-ounce cans of chopped tomatoes
1 tablespoon chopped fresh parsley
1 tablespoon torn fresh basil
1 teaspoon dried oregano
½ teaspoon sugar
Salt and freshly ground black pepper

8 ounces frozen or 1 pound fresh spinach
1 tablespoon butter
8 ounces cottage cheese
1 egg, lightly beaten
2 tablespoons heavy cream
¼ cup grated Parmesan cheese
Freshly ground black pepper
6 sheets of fresh or no-boil lasagne
1 cup grated mozzarella cheese
2 tablespoons grated Swiss cheese

Preheat the oven to 350°F. To make the tomato sauce, sauté the onion and garlic in the olive oil until softened. Add the tomato paste and sauté for 1 minute. Drain and discard the juice from the cans of tomatoes and add the tomatoes to the sautéed onion. Add all the remaining ingredients, except the salt and pepper, and simmer for 10 minutes. Season to taste.

Meanwhile, to prepare the spinach and cheese layer, cook the spinach, drain thoroughly, and then sauté in the butter for a couple of minutes. In a food processor, blend together the spinach, cottage cheese, egg, cream, and Parmesan cheese. Season with a little black pepper.

To assemble the lasagne, spread a thin layer of the tomato sauce over the base of a fairly deep ovenproof dish measuring 9 x 9 inches. Lay 2 sheets of the lasagne on top. Cover with half of the spinach mixture, a third of the mozzarella cheese, and a third of the tomato sauce. Again, lay 2 sheets of the lasagne on top, spoon the remaining spinach mixture on top, and then cover with a third of the mozzarella cheese and a third of the tomato sauce.

Lay the remaining 2 sheets of lasagne on top, cover with the remaining tomato sauce and mozzarella cheese, and then sprinkle the Swiss cheese over the top. Bake in the oven for about 25 minutes.

Linguine with Spring Vegetables

Since pasta is generally so popular with children, it's a good idea to combine it with foods that they are not so keen on eating. Here I have chosen some brightly colored diced vegetables to make a delicious sauce for linguine or spaghetti.

Makes 4 servings

8 ounces linguine
2 tablespoons vegetable oil
1 medium onion, finely chopped
1 clove garlic, crushed
1 cup finely diced carrot
½ cup finely diced sweet red pepper
1 cup finely diced zucchini
3 tomatoes, peeled, seeded, and chopped

2 scallions, finely sliced
1 chicken stock cube dissolved in
1½ cups boiling water
1½ tablespoons soy sauce
Salt and freshly ground black pepper
Freshly shaved Parmesan cheese (optional)

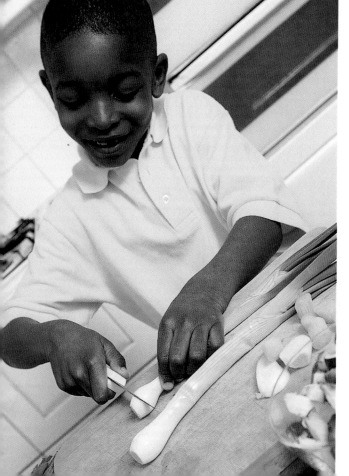

Cook the linguine in a large pot of lightly salted boiling water according to the instructions on the package. Meanwhile, heat the oil in a wok or frying pan and sauté the onion and garlic for 3 minutes, stirring occasionally. Add the carrot, red pepper, and zucchini and cook, stirring occasionally, for 4 minutes. Add the tomatoes and scallions and cook, stirring, for 2 minutes. Pour in the chicken stock and soy sauce and cook for 1 minute. Season to taste. Drain the pasta and toss with the sauce. Serve with the Parmesan cheese, if using.

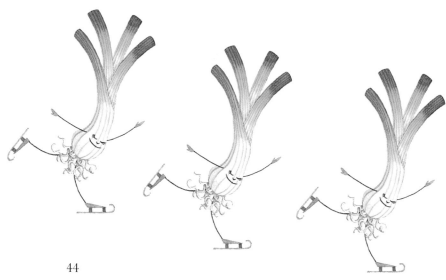

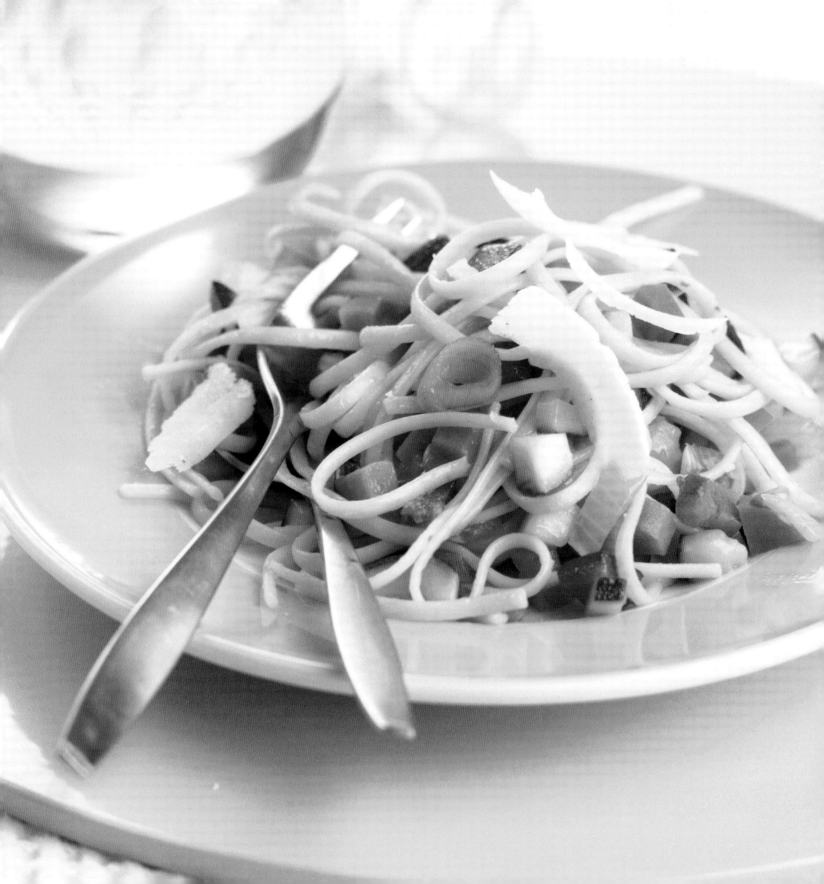

Bow-Tie Pasta with Peas and Prosciutto

Here is a simple and quick pasta dish that tends to be popular with young children. You can also add a little crème fraîche to the sauce if you like. The garlic is optional in this dish because it is especially pronounced; if you or your children aren't too keen on garlic, feel free to omit it.

Makes 2 servings

1 tablespoon olive oil
2 tablespoons butter
1 medium onion, finely chopped
1 clove garlic, crushed (optional)
¾ cup frozen peas

1 tablespoon chopped fresh parsley
½ cup chicken stock
1½ ounces prosciutto, finely diced
8 ounces bow-tie pasta
2 tablespoons grated Parmesan cheese

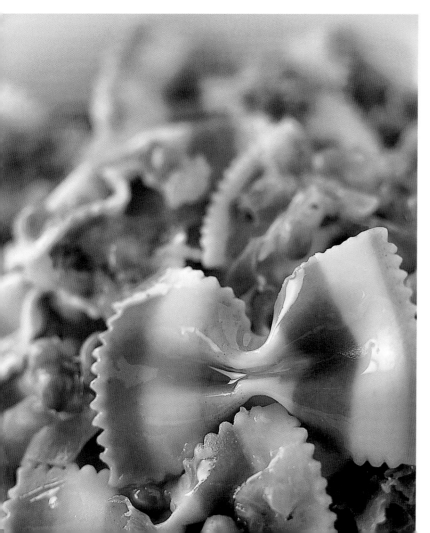

Heat the olive oil and a small amount of the butter and sauté the onion and garlic, if using, for about 8 minutes or until the onion is softened. Add the peas, cook for 1 minute, then stir in the parsley and chicken stock. Bring to a boil, then reduce the heat and cook for 4 to 5 minutes. Stir in the prosciutto.

Meanwhile, cook the pasta in a large pot of lightly salted boiling water according to the instructions on the package. Drain the pasta, return to the warm pan, add the remaining butter, and toss until it melts. Stir in the grated Parmesan cheese. Reheat the peas and prosciutto and toss with the cooked pasta. Serve with some extra grated Parmesan cheese if you wish.

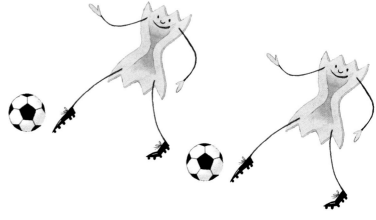

Penne with Chicken, Tomatoes, and Basil

There is a lovely mixture of flavors in this tasty chicken and pasta dish and it's very quick and easy to put together.

Makes 4 servings

8 ounces penne pasta
1 tablespoon olive oil
1 teaspoon butter
2 shallots or 1 small onion, finely chopped
2 tablespoons pine nuts
2 boneless, skinless chicken breasts,
thinly sliced into strips

¼ cup sun-dried tomatoes, drained and sliced
1 cup chicken stock
1 cup sour cream
¼ cup grated Parmesan cheese
Salt and freshly ground black pepper
2 tablespoons torn fresh basil

Cook the pasta in a large pot of lightly salted boiling water according to the instructions on the package, drain, and set aside. Meanwhile, heat the oil and butter in a large frying pan and sauté the shallots or onion and pine nuts for about 5 minutes, stirring occasionally. Add the strips of chicken and sauté, stirring occasionally, for about 5 minutes. Add the sun-dried tomatoes and cook for 1 minute.

Pour the chicken stock into the frying pan and bring to a boil. Stir in the sour cream and Parmesan cheese and season with a little salt and freshly ground black pepper. Toss the pasta with the sauce and stir in the fresh basil.

PRESERVING VITAMIN CONTENT

Many commercially frozen vegetables and fruits, such as peas, spinach, corn, and berry fruits, are frozen within 2 to 3 hours of being picked, thus ensuring that they retain their vital nutrients. In fact, fresh vegetables and fruits that have been stored for several days can sometimes contain fewer nutrients than the frozen variety.

The best method of cooking to retain maximum nutrients is steaming, microwaving, or stir-frying. Boiled broccoli retains only 35 percent of its vitamin C as opposed to 72 percent when it is steamed or microwaved. If you want to boil vegetables, cook them in a small amount of water (just enough to cover the vegetables) and do not overcook. Scrub or wash fruit and vegetables rather than peeling them, as most of the nutrients lie just beneath the surface. When possible, try to buy organic fruit and vegetables. Vitamin C dissolves in water, so avoid standing fruit and vegetables in water.

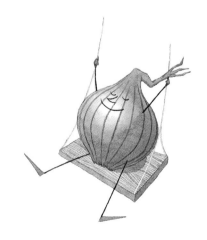

Vegetable Tagliatelle

This is a lovely light sauce with vegetables and cherry tomatoes that can be served with almost any kind of pasta. It is a particularly good summer pasta recipe.

Makes 4 servings

8 ounces tagliatelle
1 tablespoon olive oil
1 medium onion, finely chopped
1 clove garlic, finely chopped
1 small yellow pepper, cut into strips
1 cup broccoli florets
1 medium zucchini, sliced diagonally and cut into semicircles

½ cup light sour cream
½ cup vegetable stock
8 cherry tomatoes, halved
¾ cup grated Parmesan cheese
Salt and freshly ground black pepper

Cook the tagliatelle in a large pot of lightly salted boiling water according to the directions on the package. Meanwhile, heat the olive oil in a heavy-bottomed saucepan and sauté the onion and garlic for 1 minute. Add the yellow pepper, broccoli, and zucchini and sauté for about 8 minutes or until tender. Stir in the sour cream and vegetable stock and bring to a simmer. Stir in the cherry tomatoes and simmer for 1 minute, then stir in the Parmesan cheese and season to taste. Drain the tagliatelle and toss with the sauce. Serve with extra Parmesan cheese to sprinkle on top if you wish.

Turkey Bolognese

A tasty, quick, and easy sauce for pasta. You can also make this with chopped chicken.

Makes 4 servings

1 large onion, finely chopped
1 clove garlic, finely chopped
1 small sweet red pepper, finely diced
2 tablespoons vegetable oil
1 pound ground turkey
1 medium carrot, peeled and grated
One 14-ounce can of chopped tomatoes

1 chicken stock cube dissolved in 1 cup boiling water
1 tablespoon ketchup
1 tablespoon chopped fresh sage or ½ teaspoon dried sage
1½ teaspoons chopped fresh thyme or
¼ teaspoon dried thyme
Salt and freshly ground black pepper
12 ounces spaghetti or penne

Sauté the onion, garlic, and red pepper in the vegetable oil for 3 to 4 minutes. Add the turkey and stir until it changes color, breaking up any lumps with a fork. Add the remaining ingredients, bring to a boil, and simmer, stirring occasionally, for 30 minutes. Meanwhile, cook the pasta in lightly salted boiling water according to the instructions on the package. Drain, and toss with the sauce.

Tagliatelle with Shrimp and Vegetables

I often make this for my own supper, as two of my favorite foods are pasta and shrimp. It also makes an excellent vegetable pasta dish without the shrimp.

Makes 4 servings

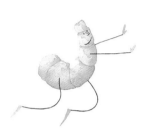

8 ounces tagliatelle
1 teaspoon butter plus 2 tablespoons butter
3 cups chicken stock
1 teaspoon lemon juice
1 cup small cauliflower florets
1 medium carrot, peeled
and cut into matchsticks
2 ounces green beans, trimmed
1 small onion, finely chopped

1 small clove garlic, crushed
4 small zucchini, cut into matchsticks
6 ounces cooked and peeled large or jumbo
shrimp, either fresh or frozen and defrosted
1 tablespoon chopped fresh parsley
Salt and freshly ground black pepper
1 tablespoon cornstarch
¼ cup light sour cream
¼ cup grated Parmesan cheese

Cook the tagliatelle in a large pot of lightly salted boiling water according to the instructions on the package. When it is just tender, drain, add the 1 teaspoon butter, and toss the warm pasta with the butter. Set aside.

Put the chicken stock and lemon juice into a saucepan, bring to a boil, add the cauliflower, carrot, and green beans, and cook over medium heat for about 6 minutes or until the vegetables are just tender. Strain the vegetables, reserving the stock for later use.

Melt the 2 tablespoons butter in a frying pan, add the onion and garlic, and sauté for 3 to 4 minutes. Add the zucchini and continue to cook for 3 to 4 minutes. Cut the shrimp in half and add the shrimp together with the parsley and the drained vegetables. Lightly season, and cook for 2 to 3 minutes or until heated through.

Mix a little of the reserved stock with the cornstarch and heat the remaining stock in a saucepan. Mix the cornstarch liquid into the remaining stock and cook, stirring, for about 3 minutes or until the stock thickens. Remove from the heat and stir in the sour cream. Toss the tagliatelle with the vegetables and sauce until well mixed. Serve with the grated Parmesan cheese.

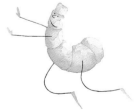

Scarlett's Pasta

This pasta dish is a great favorite with my children, especially Scarlett, who loves both pasta and salami. You can also use sliced sausage instead of salami if you prefer.

Makes 4 servings

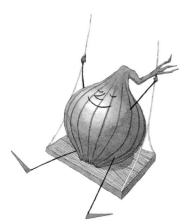

2 shallots, finely chopped
½ small sweet red pepper, chopped
1 tablespoon olive oil
One 14-ounce can of chopped tomatoes, drained
¾ cup chicken stock

8 ounces pasta (any shape)
1 tablespoon torn fresh basil
1 tablespoon grated Parmesan cheese
14 ounces salami, cut into strips
Salt and freshly ground black pepper

Sauté the shallots and red pepper in the olive oil for about 5 minutes or until softened. Stir in the tomatoes and sauté for 2 minutes, then add the stock and simmer for about 10 minutes. Meanwhile, cook the pasta in lightly salted boiling water according to the instructions on the package. When the vegetables are cooked, stir in the basil, Parmesan cheese, and salami, heat through, and season to taste. Drain the pasta and toss with the sauce.

VERY QUICK AND EASY PASTA SAUCE

For a simple sauce that tastes delicious, simmer 2 cups light cream with 4 tablespoons butter and seasoning. Toss with freshly cooked pasta such as tagliatelle and fresh Parmesan cheese.

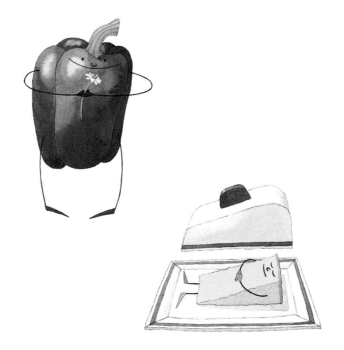

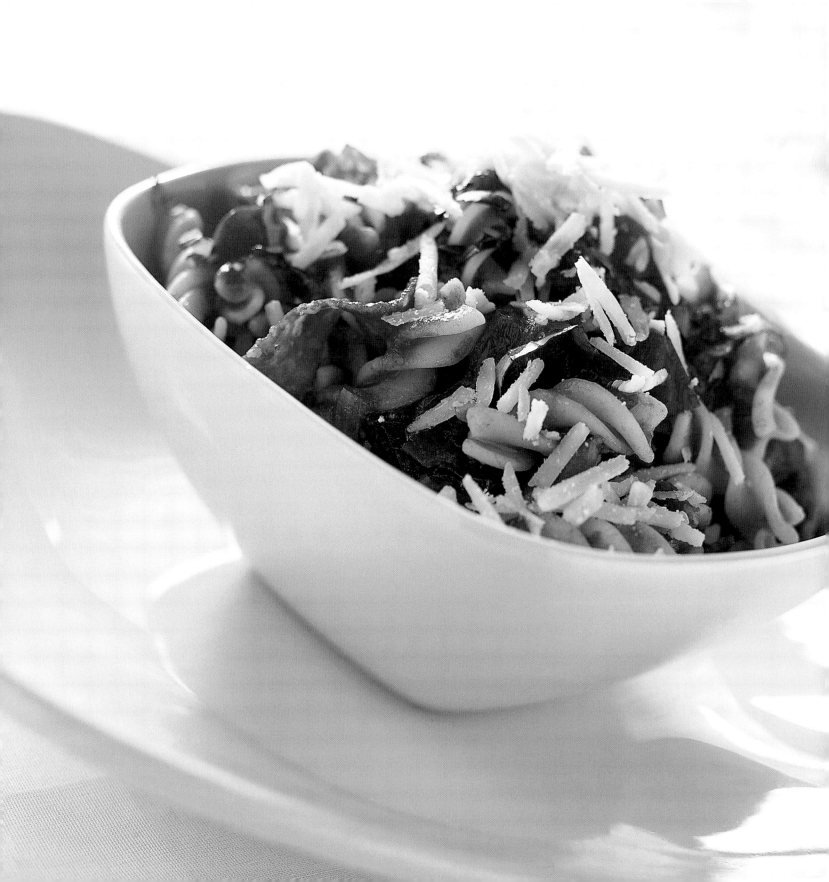

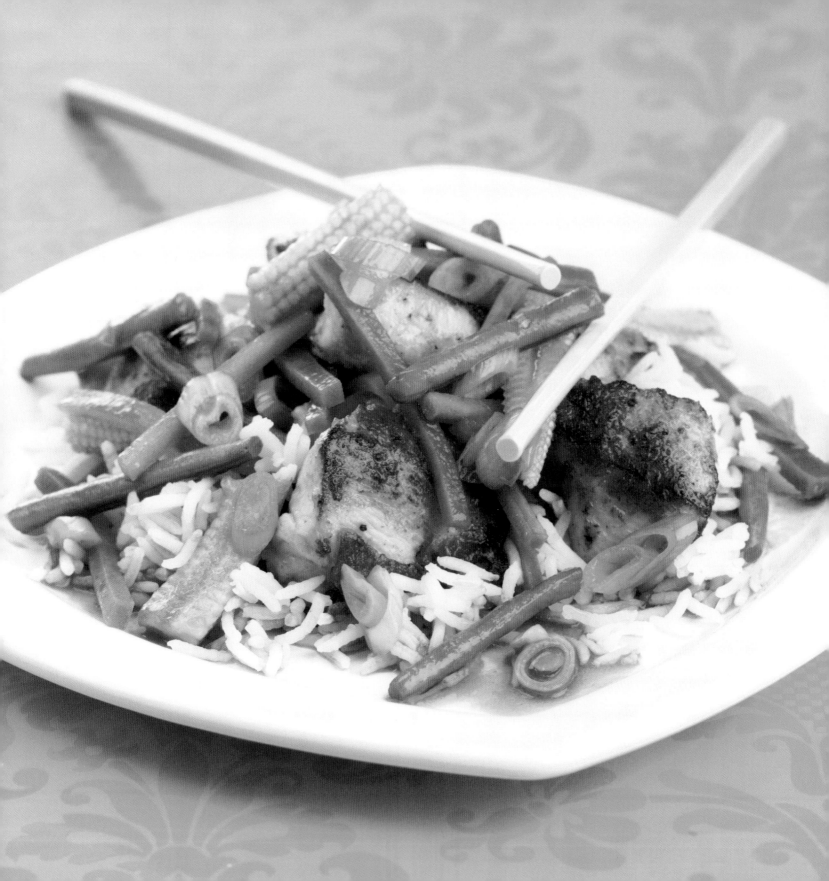

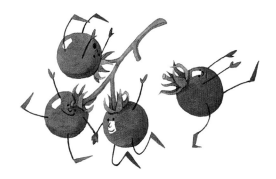

Poultry

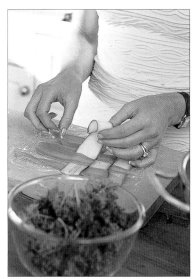

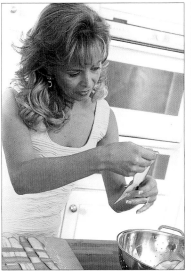

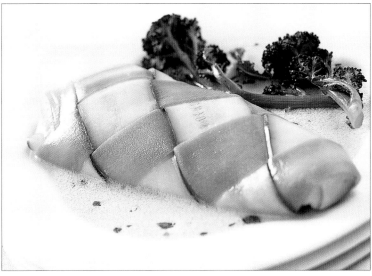

Chicken Balls in Sweet-and-Sour Sauce

The grated apple adds a delicious flavor. You can also use ground beef to make the meatballs.

Makes 4 servings

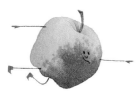

1 large Granny Smith apple, peeled and grated
2 large boneless, skinless chicken breasts,
cut into chunks
1 medium onion, finely chopped
1 tablespoon chopped fresh parsley
½ cup fresh white bread crumbs
2 teaspoons chicken stock, dissolved in
1 teaspoon boiling water
Salt and freshly ground black pepper
All-purpose flour for coating
Vegetable oil for frying

Sweet-and-Sour Sauce
1 medium onion, finely chopped
1 small sweet red pepper, seeded and chopped
1½ tablespoons vegetable oil
One 14-ounce can of chopped tomatoes
1 tablespoon tomato paste
½ cup pineapple juice
1 teaspoon light brown sugar
1 teaspoon malt vinegar
1 teaspoon soy sauce
Freshly ground black pepper

Using your hands, squeeze out some of the excess liquid from the grated apple. Combine the chicken, onion, parsley, crumbs, apple, and stock and chop in a food processor for a few seconds. Season with a little salt and pepper. With your hands, form into about 20 balls, roll in the flour, and panfry until lightly golden, about 10 minutes. For the sauce, sauté the onion and red pepper in the oil until softened. Add the rest of the ingredients, bring to a boil, and simmer, covered, for 15 minutes. Pour over the balls and serve with rice.

Tasty Satay Chicken Skewers

Makes 8 skewers

Marinade
1 tablespoon soy sauce
1½ tablespoons lime juice
1 tablespoon smooth peanut butter
1 tablespoon honey
½ teaspoon mild curry powder

1 clove garlic, crushed

2 boneless, skinless chicken breasts,
each cut lengthwise into 4 strips
2 tablespoons coconut milk
Chopped fresh coriander, to garnish (optional)

Combine the marinade ingredients. Place the chicken strips in the marinade and leave for at least 30 minutes. Remove the chicken and reserve the marinade. Thread the chicken strips onto presoaked bamboo skewers. Brush a griddle pan with a little oil and heat until hot. Sear the outside of the chicken, then reduce the heat and cook for 3 to 4 minutes on each side or until cooked through. You can also broil the skewers for 4 to 5 minutes on each side. To make the sauce, put the reserved marinade into a small saucepan. Bring to a boil, add the coconut milk, and cook for 1 minute. Scatter the chopped coriander, if using, over the skewers and serve with the sauce.

Annabel's Tasty Chicken Skewers

These skewers can also be interspersed with some vegetables, such as chunks of sweet red pepper, onion, or some button mushrooms. Brush the vegetables with the marinade before cooking the skewers. Alternatively, make the skewers with chicken only and serve with boiled rice into which stir-fried chopped onion and diced red and yellow peppers have been stirred to give the rice both color and flavor.

Makes 4 servings

¼ cup soy sauce
⅓ cup light brown sugar
1 tablespoon lime or lemon juice
1 tablespoon vegetable oil

1 clove garlic, crushed
4 boneless, skinless chicken breasts, cut into chunks

Put the soy sauce and sugar into a small saucepan and gently heat, stirring until the sugar has dissolved. Remove from the heat and stir in the lime or lemon juice, vegetable oil, and garlic. Marinate the chicken for at least 1 hour or overnight. Soak 8 bamboo skewers in water to prevent them from getting scorched. Thread the chunks of chicken onto the skewers and cook under a preheated broiler for 4 to 5 minutes on each side, basting occasionally with the marinade until cooked through.

Teriyaki Chicken Skewers

Marinated chicken skewers make an easy to prepare and very tasty meal. They are also good cooked on a barbecue. It is also good to make these using chicken thighs instead of chicken breasts. The dark meat of the chicken has more flavor and is lovely and moist; it also provides twice as much iron and zinc as the white meat.

Makes 4 servings

Marinade
2 tablespoons soy sauce
1 teaspoon sesame oil
1 tablespoon rice wine vinegar
3 teaspoons honey
1 clove garlic, crushed

½-inch piece of gingerroot, peeled and grated (optional)

4 small boneless, skinless chicken breasts or 4 large boneless chicken thighs

Combine the ingredients for the marinade. Cut each chicken breast into 4 strips and marinate for at least 30 minutes. Soak eight bamboo skewers in water to prevent them from scorching. Thread the chicken strips onto the skewers in the shape of a wiggly snake, then cook under a preheated broiler for 4 to 5 minutes on each side. If using chicken thighs, remove the skin, cut the flesh into bite-size cubes, and trim away any fat. Thread the chicken cubes onto the skewers.

Teriyaki Chicken Skewers are shown on pages 56–57.

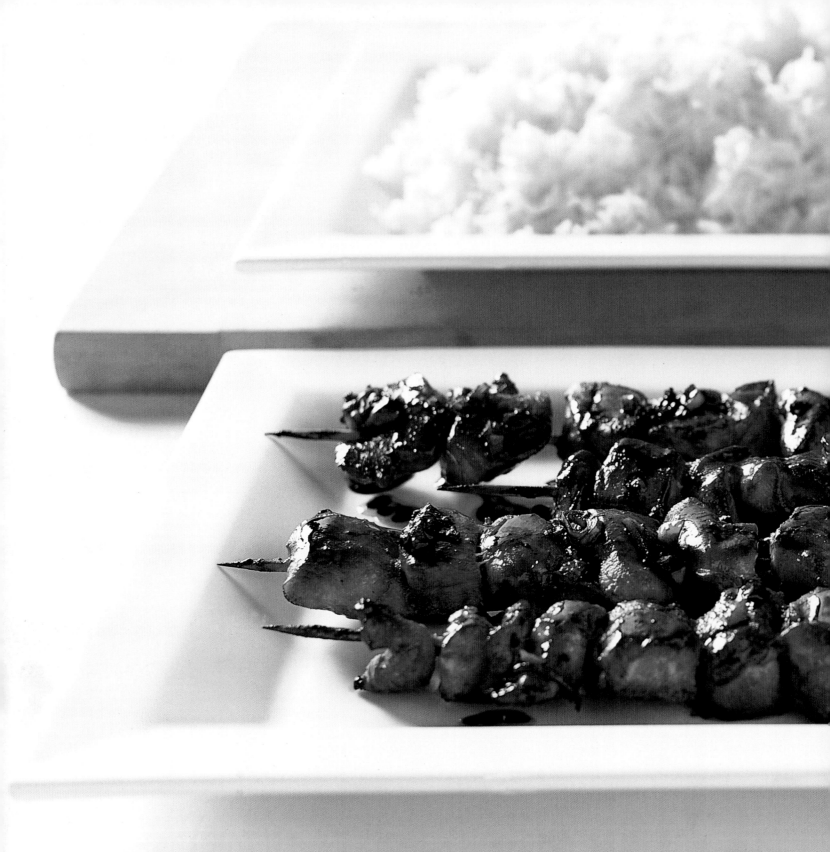

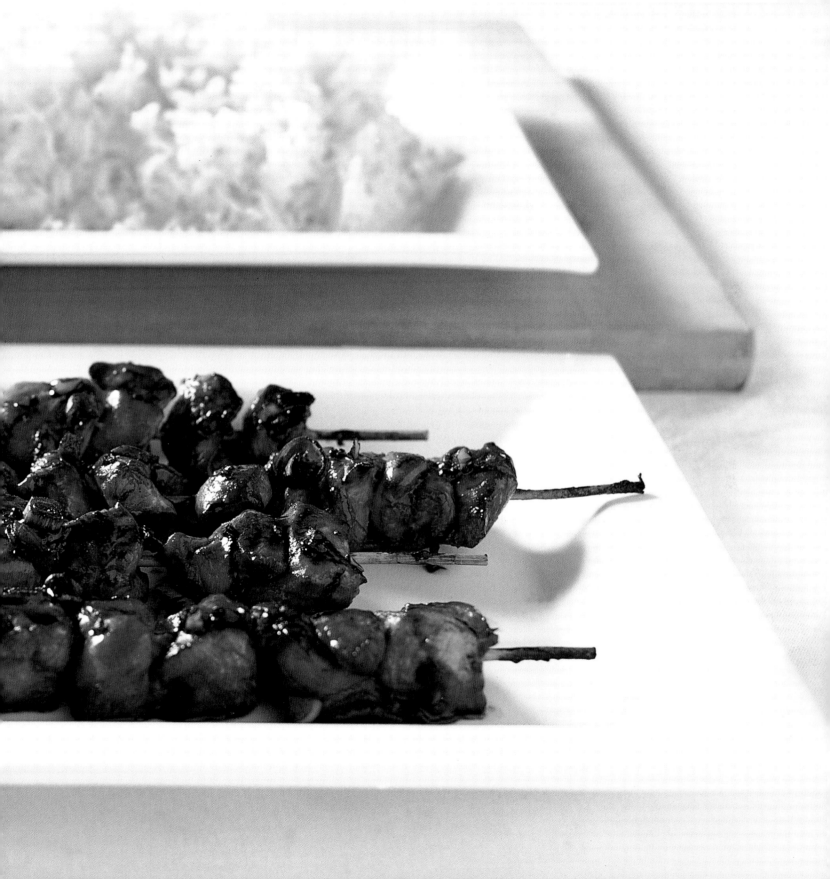

Chicken Piccata

Here are tender breasts of chicken cooked in a delicious, quick, and easy to prepare Chinese-style sauce.

**Makes 2
servings**

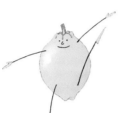

2 boneless, skinless chicken breasts

Marinade
1 tablespoon lemon juice
1 tablespoon water
1 tablespoon finely chopped onion

All-purpose flour
Salt and freshly ground black pepper
2 tablespoons vegetable oil

Sauce
1 cup chicken stock
2 teaspoons soy sauce
1 teaspoon sesame oil
1 tablespoon sugar
1 teaspoon cider vinegar
1 tablespoon cornstarch
Ground white pepper
1 scallion, thinly sliced

Rinse the chicken and pat dry with paper towels. Place the chicken breasts under a layer of plastic wrap and, using the flat side of a meat mallet, pound until quite thin. Remove the plastic wrap, cut each breast in half, and place the chicken in a shallow dish. Mix together the lemon juice and water, add the chopped onion, and marinate the chicken for 30 minutes. Remove the chicken pieces and discard the marinade. Dip the chicken in seasoned flour. Heat the vegetable oil in a frying pan or wok and sauté the chicken for about 5 minutes on each side or until lightly browned and cooked through. Meanwhile, put all the ingredients for the sauce into a saucepan and bring to a boil. Cook over medium heat, stirring until thickened. Drain away any excess oil from the pan in which the chicken was cooked, pour the sauce over the cooked chicken, and heat through.

Chicken Fajitas

Children can eat these chicken fajitas with their hands. Wrap the fajitas up in colorful napkins.
They are also good cold in a lunch box.

**Makes 3 large
or
4 small tortillas**

1 tablespoon olive oil
1 small clove garlic, crushed
½ cup sliced red onion
½ sweet red pepper, cored, seeded,
and cut into strips
1 boneless, skinless chicken breast,
cut into strips
½ red chile, finely chopped

½ teaspoon balsamic vinegar
One 8-ounce can of chopped tomatoes
1 tablespoon chopped fresh oregano or
1 teaspoon dried oregano
Salt and freshly ground black pepper
3 large or 4 small tortillas
Shredded lettuce
3 tablespoons sour cream

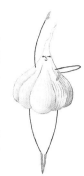

eat the oil in a wok or frying pan, add the garlic, onion, and sweet red pepper and stir-fry for 3 minutes. Add the chicken and chile and stir-fry for another 3 minutes. Add the balsamic vinegar and cook for a few seconds, then add the chopped tomatoes, oregano, and seasoning. Cook for about 4 minutes or until the mixture has thickened.

To assemble, heat the tortillas in the microwave or frying pan according to the package instructions. Place some of the chicken mixture along the center of each tortilla, add some shredded lettuce and a little sour cream, and roll up. Serve immediately.

Chicken Karmel

This sweet-and-sour chicken is a great favorite with children, and my family loves it. Serve with white rice. To make eating fun, you can buy child-friendly plastic chopsticks that are joined at the top so that they only need to be squeezed together to pick up food. This dish would be perfect for these, as everything is cut into bite-size pieces. If your child isn't keen on green beans or baby corn, use different vegetables or simply omit them (see photograph, page 52).

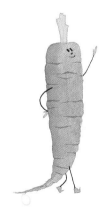

Makes 4 servings

Batter
1 egg yolk
1½ tablespoons cornstarch
1 tablespoon milk

¼ cup vegetable oil
2 boneless, skinless chicken breasts,
cut into bite-size cubes

Sweet-and-Sour Sauce
1 tablespoon soy sauce
2 tablespoons ketchup

2 tablespoons rice wine vinegar
2 tablespoons superfine sugar
½ teaspoon sesame oil

1 medium carrot, peeled and
cut into matchsticks
4 canned whole baby corn, sliced in half
lengthwise, then in half across
2 ounces thin green beans, trimmed and
cut in half
2 scallions, finely sliced
Salt and freshly ground black pepper

In a small bowl, beat together the egg yolk, cornstarch, and milk to make a thin batter. Heat 2 tablespoons of the oil in a wok, dip the chicken into the batter, then fry for 3 to 4 minutes, until golden. Remove from the wok and set aside.

Meanwhile, mix together all the ingredients for the sweet-and-sour sauce. Heat the remaining 2 tablespoons vegetable oil in a wok and stir-fry the carrot, baby corn, and green beans for 2 minutes. Add the sauce, bring to a boil, and cook for 2 minutes. Remove from the heat and stir in the scallions. Add the chicken to the vegetables and heat through. Season to taste.

Turkey Burgers

These turkey burgers can also be eaten sandwiched between a bun and layered with lettuce and tomato sauce.

Makes 12 burgers

1 pound turkey breast, roughly chopped, or ground turkey
1 medium onion, finely chopped
1 tablespoon chopped fresh thyme or oregano or ½ teaspoon dried thyme or oregano
1 tablespoon chopped fresh parsley
1 apple, peeled and grated (squeeze out excess juice)

½ cup fresh white bread crumbs
1 chicken stock cube dissolved in 1½ tablespoons boiling water
1 teaspoon Worcestershire sauce
Salt and freshly ground black pepper
½ cup all-purpose flour
2 eggs, lightly beaten
Vegetable oil for frying

Mix together the turkey, onion, herbs, and apple. Chop for a few seconds in a food processor. Place the mixture in a large bowl and stir in about half the crumbs, the stock, and Worcestershire sauce and season to taste. Form the mixture into 12 burgers. Dip the burgers in the flour, then in the eggs, and coat with the remaining bread crumbs. Panfry the burgers for about 4 minutes on each side or until cooked through.

Annabel's Tasty Beefburgers

These tasty burgers can be made with beef, lamb, or chicken.

Makes 10 burgers

½ sweet red pepper, cored, seeded, and chopped
1 medium onion, finely chopped
1 tablespoon vegetable oil
1 pound lean ground beef or lamb
1 tablespoon chopped fresh parsley
1 beef stock cube, finely crumbled
1 apple, peeled and grated
½ lightly beaten egg
¼ cup fresh white bread crumbs

1½ teaspoons Worcestershire sauce
Salt and freshly ground black pepper
All-purpose flour

Sauce
2 tablespoons hoisin sauce
1 tablespoon water
1 teaspoon sesame oil
Vegetable oil for frying

Fry the red pepper and half the onion in the vegetable oil for about 5 minutes or until softened. In a mixing bowl, combine the sautéed onion and pepper and the remaining chopped raw onion with the rest of the burger ingredients. With floured hands, form into 10 burgers. Combine sauce ingredients. Panfry the burgers over high heat to brown and seal, then lower the heat and cook for 3 to 4 minutes. Brush the sauce on top of the burgers. Turn and cook for 3 minutes. Brush again, turn, and cook for 1 minute. Or barbecue: brush with sauce and cook for 1 minute on each side.

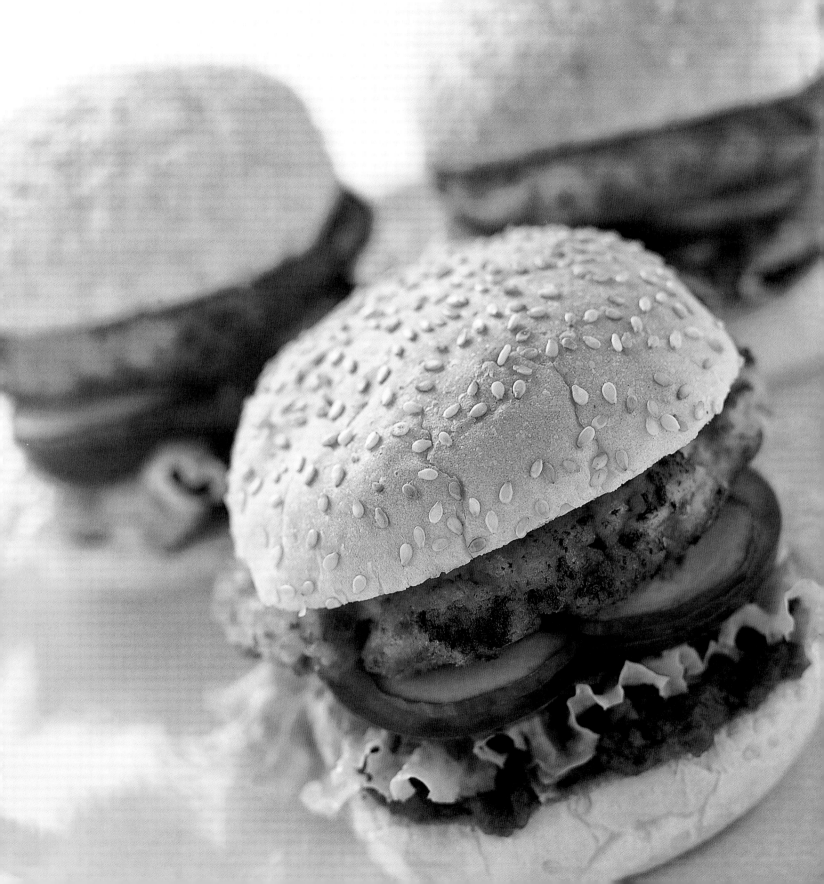

Fruity Curried Chicken

A mild, deliciously flavored chicken curry. This is a recipe that my mother used to make for me when I was a child. I like a pretty tame curry, but you can always make it more fiery by using a medium or hot curry powder. Serve with plain rice and pappadams.

Makes 6 servings

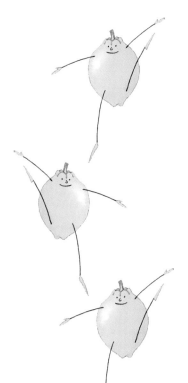

1 chicken, cut into about 8 pieces
All-purpose flour
Salt and freshly ground black pepper
Vegetable oil
2 medium onions, chopped
2 tablespoons mild curry powder
6 tablespoons tomato paste
3 cups chicken stock

1 medium cooking apple (Granny Smith or Golden Delicious), peeled and thinly sliced
1 large carrot, peeled and thinly sliced
2 lemon slices
½ cup raisins
1 bay leaf
1 teaspoon brown sugar

Preheat the oven to 350°F. Trim any fat from the chicken and remove some of the skin. Coat the chicken with seasoned flour. Fry in vegetable oil until lightly golden, then drain on paper towels and place in a casserole dish. Heat 2 tablespoons of vegetable oil in a frying pan and sauté the onions for about 10 minutes or until softened but not colored. Stir in the curry powder and tomato paste and continue to cook for 2 to 3 minutes. Stir in 2 tablespoons of flour and stir in 2 cups of the stock.

Add the sliced apple, carrot, lemon slices, raisins, bay leaf, brown sugar, and the remaining 1 cup stock. Season with salt and pepper. Pour the sauce over the chicken in the casserole, cover, and bake in the oven for 1 hour. Remove the lemon slices and bay leaf, take the chicken off the bone, and cut into pieces.

Chicken and Potato Pancake

This pancake is deliciously thick, golden, and crispy with a soft, succulent center. The recipe can be varied by adding other vegetables such as grated zucchini or chopped sweet peppers. I make it in an 8-inch frying pan and my children enjoy cutting their own slices—it can be eaten either hot or cold.

Makes 4 servings

1 boneless, skinless chicken breast,
cut into pieces, or
1 cup diced cooked chicken
2 cups chicken or vegetable stock
1 baking potato, peeled and grated
1 medium onion, grated

2 tablespoons frozen peas
1 small egg, lightly beaten
1 tablespoon all-purpose flour
Salt and freshly ground black pepper
2 tablespoons vegetable oil

Poach the chicken breast in the stock until cooked through, 10 to 15 minutes. Press out the liquid from the grated potato and combine the potato with the onion, frozen peas, egg, and flour and season lightly with some salt and freshly ground black pepper. Dice the chicken and add it to the vegetable mixture.

Heat 1 tablespoon of the oil in an 8-inch frying pan, tilt the pan so that the oil coats the sides, and press the mixture into the pan. Fry for about 5 minutes or until browned. Turn the pancake onto a plate. Heat the remaining 1 tablespoon oil and brown the pancake on the other side for about 7 minutes. Cut into wedges and serve.

Finger-Licking Chicken Drumsticks

Chicken drumsticks tend to be very popular with children and are good either hot or cold. This tasty marinade gives them a wonderful flavor and they can be prepared the day before, refrigerated, and then wrapped in foil for your child's lunch box. Always take care to cook chicken right through to avoid food poisoning.

Makes 4 servings

Marinade
1½ tablespoons cider or white wine vinegar
¼ cup tomato sauce
2 tablespoons honey
1½ teaspoons Dijon mustard
1½ teaspoons Worcestershire sauce
1½ teaspoons vegetable oil

4 large drumsticks

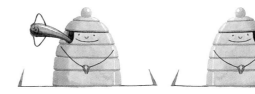

Mix all the ingredients for the marinade together in a bowl. Skin the drumsticks, make 2 to 3 slashes in the flesh, and add to the marinade, turning a few times to make sure that they are well coated. Cover and refrigerate for at least 2 hours or overnight.

Preheat the oven to 425°F. Arrange the drumsticks in a shallow roasting pan and pour over the marinade. Cook for 35 to 40 minutes or until cooked through, basting occasionally with the sauce.

Basket-Weave Chicken Breasts

The bright orange and green basket-weave pattern made by the carrot and zucchini strips looks sensational wrapped around these stuffed chicken breasts. This is a great dish to make for a dinner party. They are surprisingly easy to make and children will love to help weave the vegetable strips together. If your child prefers, you can stuff the chicken breasts with some cheese and ham.

Makes 2 servings

1 large carrot, peeled
1 large zucchini
1 shallot, finely chopped
1½ teaspoons vegetable oil and a little butter
¾ cup chopped button mushrooms
1 teaspoon chopped fresh parsley
Squeeze of lemon juice
1 tablespoon bread crumbs
Salt and freshly ground black pepper

2 large boneless, skinless chicken breasts

Tarragon Sauce
¼ cup chicken stock
1½ tablespoons lime or lemon juice
4 tablespoons cold butter, cut into cubes
1½ teaspoons chopped fresh tarragon
2 tablespoons heavy cream
Salt and freshly ground black pepper

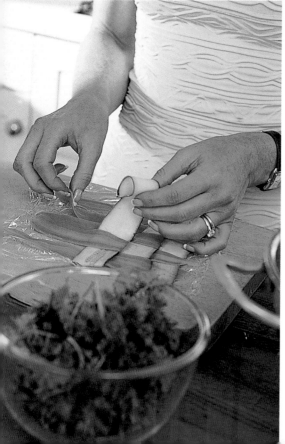

Using a potato peeler, cut the carrot and zucchini lengthwise into long thin strips. Blanch them in boiling water for just under 1 minute and place on paper towels to dry.

To prepare the mushroom stuffing, sauté the shallot in the oil and butter until softened, add the chopped mushrooms, and cook for 3 to 4 minutes. Add the parsley, lemon juice, and bread crumbs and cook for 2 minutes. Season to taste. Cut a slit in each of the chicken breasts to form a pocket and stuff with the mushroom mixture. Season the chicken.

Place 5 strips of zucchini horizontally quite close together on top of a piece of plastic wrap just big enough to wrap around the chicken breast. Weave 5 strips of carrot vertically through the zucchini strips to make a basket-weave pattern. Wrap the plastic wrap and woven vegetables around the chicken breasts to form a parcel. Cook in a steamer for about 20 minutes or until cooked through.

To make the sauce, put the stock and lime or lemon juice in a small saucepan and bring to a boil. Remove from the heat and whisk in the butter. Stir in the tarragon and cream and season to taste. Pour some of the sauce onto each plate, remove the plastic wrap, and place a chicken breast on top of the sauce.

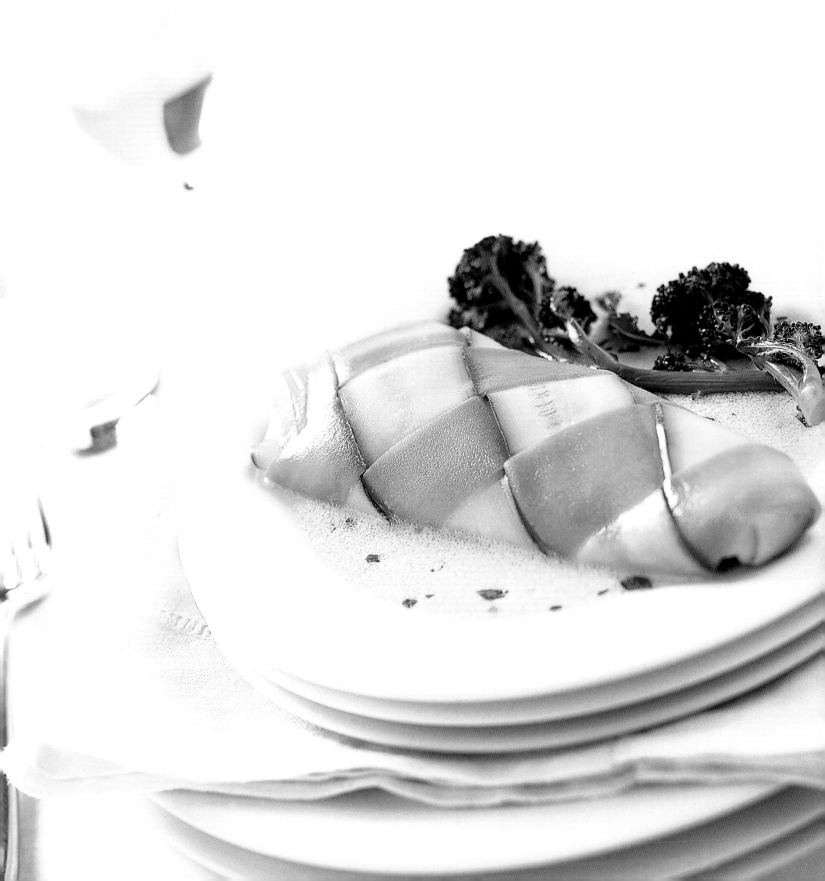

Chicken Burgers with Zucchini and Apple

The grated apples and zucchini give these burgers a lovely moist flavor. They are a great favorite with the whole family and also make a good standby in the freezer.
They are good served in a bun with lettuce and tomato sauce or simply with baked beans.

Makes 12 burgers

2 boneless, skinless chicken breasts, chopped
1 tablespoon chopped fresh parsley
1 medium onion, finely chopped
2 apples, peeled and grated
2 medium or 1 large zucchini, grated
1 chicken stock cube, crumbled

Salt and freshly ground black pepper
¾ cup all-purpose flour
2 eggs, lightly beaten
1 cup bread crumbs
Vegetable oil for frying

Place the chicken, parsley, and onion in a food processor and chop for a few seconds on pulse. Squeeze the excess moisture from the apples and zucchini, and mix into the chicken together with the crumbled stock cube and a little salt and freshly ground black pepper. Using your hands, form into burgers. Coat in the flour, then in the beaten eggs, and coat with the bread crumbs. Heat the oil in a large frying pan and sauté the burgers until golden, about 6 minutes on each side.

Terrific Turkey Schnitzels

These turkey schnitzels are a great favorite and quick to cook. I like to serve them with spaghettini (very thin spaghetti) and tomato sauce, preferably homemade (see page 38). If you can't find turkey cutlets, you can substitute chicken breasts pounded quite thin. If you don't have sesame seeds, use ½ cup bread crumbs instead. It will improve the flavor if you marinate the turkey in lemon juice and garlic before coating with the bread crumbs and sesame seeds.

Makes 2 servings

2 turkey cutlets, about 6 ounces each,
or 2 boneless, skinless chicken breasts

Marinade
1 tablespoon olive oil
2 tablespoons lemon juice
1 small clove garlic, thinly sliced

All-purpose flour
Salt and freshly ground black pepper

1 egg
1 tablespoon milk
⅓ cup bread crumbs
2 tablespoons sesame seeds
1 tablespoon finely chopped fresh parsley
1 tablespoon mixed chopped fresh herbs,
such as chives, sage, thyme, rosemary,
or 1½ teaspoons dried herbs
1 tablespoon vegetable oil
2 tablespoons butter

TIP

You can also use this marinade to marinate chicken breasts, and then cook them under a preheated broiler or on a griddle with a sprinkling of fresh herbs and some sea salt.

Place the turkey cutlets or chicken breasts between sheets of plastic wrap and pound them with the smooth side of a mallet until very thin. Mix together the ingredients for the marinade and marinate the meat for at least 30 minutes. Remove from the marinade and season the flour with salt and freshly ground black pepper. Lightly beat the egg with the milk.

Mix together the bread crumbs, sesame seeds, parsley, and herbs. Toss each turkey cutlet in the seasoned flour, shake off the excess, dip into the egg mixture, and roll in the bread crumb mixture. Sauté in a mixture of vegetable oil and butter for about 5 minutes, turning halfway through, until lightly golden. These taste good with a little fresh lemon juice squeezed over them, so serve with half a lemon if you like.

Nasi Goreng

This is a delicious Indonesian recipe flavored with peanuts and a mild curry sauce.

Makes 6 servings

2 boneless, skinless chicken breasts, diced

Marinade
2 tablespoons soy sauce
1½ teaspoons sesame oil
1 tablespoon dark brown sugar

2½ tablespoons vegetable oil
1½ teaspoons sesame oil
8 canned whole baby corn, cut into pieces
1 sweet red pepper, cored, seeded, and finely chopped

1 large onion, finely chopped
1½ cups long-grain rice
2 teaspoons mild curry powder
½ teaspoon ground turmeric
3 cups chicken stock
1 cup frozen peas
3 scallions, finely sliced
1 tablespoon molasses or dark brown sugar
½ cup finely chopped roasted peanuts
Salt and freshly ground black pepper

Marinate the chicken in the soy sauce, sesame oil, and sugar for 30 minutes, then strain the chicken and reserve the marinade. Heat 1 tablespoon of the vegetable oil in a wok and stir-fry the chicken for 2 minutes, then set aside. Heat the sesame oil and 1½ teaspoons of the vegetable oil and stir-fry the corn and red pepper for 3 minutes. Heat the remaining 1 tablespoon vegetable oil in a saucepan and sauté the onion for 3 minutes. Add the rice and cook for 1 minute, stirring to make sure that all the grains are coated. Stir in the curry powder and turmeric and cook for 30 seconds, then add the chicken stock and the reserved marinade from the chicken. Bring to a boil and cook over high heat for about 6 minutes, then lower the heat and cook for 6 minutes, stirring often so that the rice does not stick to the bottom of the pan. Add the frozen peas, scallions, molasses or dark brown sugar, chopped peanuts, cooked vegetables, and chicken and cook, stirring, for 2 minutes. Season to taste.

Teddy Bear Chicken Burgers

The apple brings out a succulent flavor in these chicken burgers. Shaping them into teddy bear faces is easy and quick and will add oodles of child appeal (see photograph).

Makes 6 teddy bears

4 boneless, skinless chicken breasts
1 leek, white part only, very finely chopped
1 apple, cored, but not peeled, and diced
3 to 4 fresh sage leaves, chopped,
or 1 teaspoon dried sage
1 chicken stock cube, finely crumbled
½ lightly beaten egg
½ cup fresh white bread crumbs
3 tablespoons vegetable oil

Decoration
Carrot
Peas
Olives
Sweet red pepper
Apple

Chop the chicken breasts in a food processor for a few seconds. Transfer the chicken to a mixing bowl and stir in the remaining ingredients except the vegetable oil. Form into 6 teddy bear shapes about ¾ inch thick and 3½ inches across. Sauté in the vegetable oil for 12 to 15 minutes, turning halfway through, or until golden and cooked through. Decorate with eyes, nose, and a mouth.

Easy Yakitori Chicken

In Japan, yakitori bars are popular places to meet, eat, and socialize. For extra flavor you can marinate the chicken in the sauce before cooking. You can also add other vegetables such as peppers or mushrooms to the skewers if you wish.

Makes 4 skewers

3 tablespoons sake or sherry
3 tablespoons soy sauce
3 tablespoons mirin
1 tablespoon sugar
2 boneless, skinless chicken breasts
or 8 boneless chicken thighs

2 large scallions or 1 leek, white part only,
cut into 1-inch lengths
1 tablespoon vegetable oil

Soak 4 bamboo skewers in water. Put the sake or sherry, soy sauce, mirin, and sugar into a small saucepan, bring to a boil, and simmer for 6 to 8 minutes or until syrupy. Cut the chicken breasts into chunks and thread onto the skewers alternately with the scallions or leek. Stir the vegetable oil into the sauce and brush the chicken liberally with the sauce. Cook under a preheated broiler for 4 to 5 minutes on each side or until the chicken is cooked through.

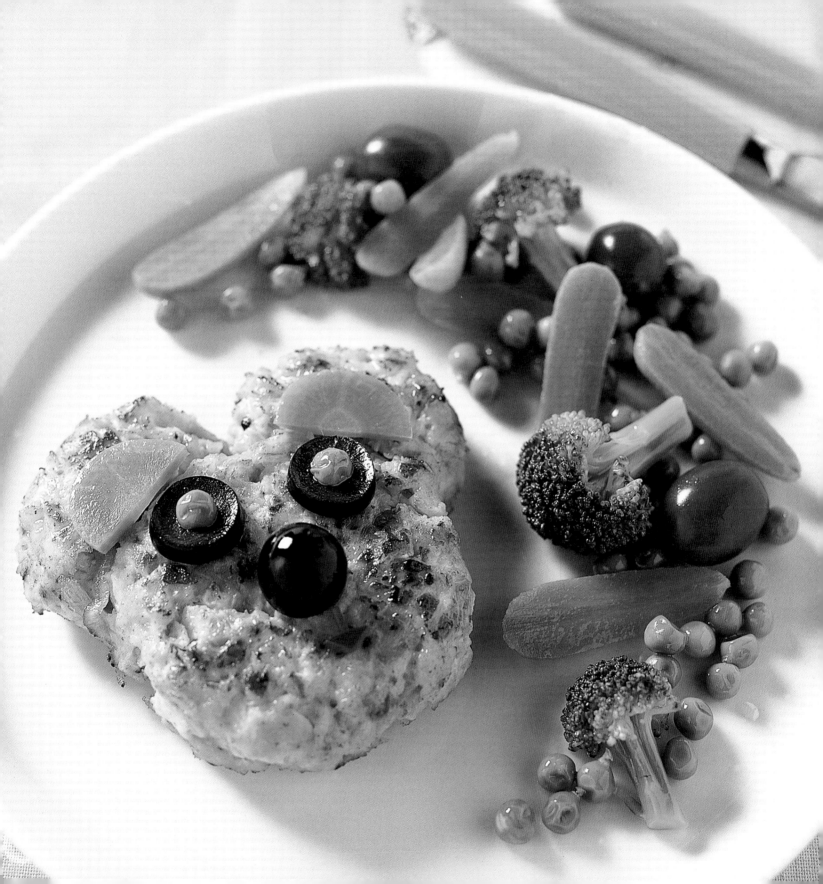

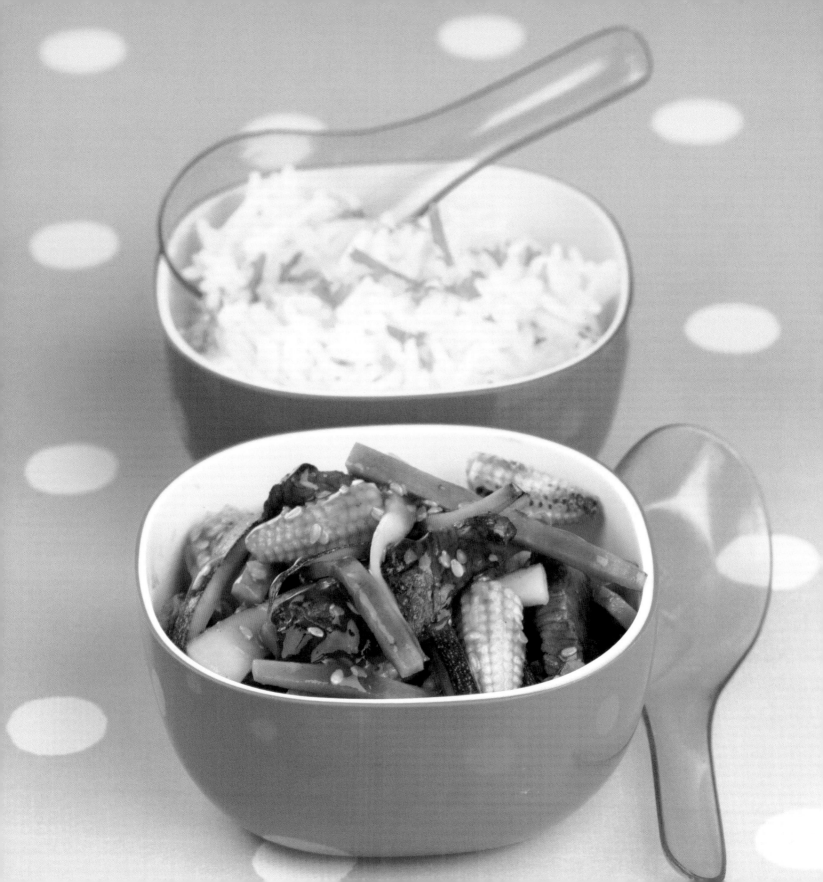

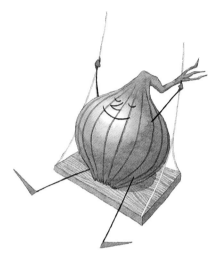

Meat

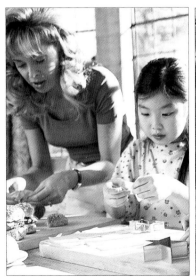

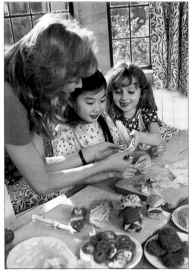

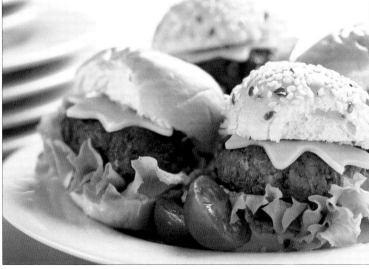

Meatballs with Sweet-and-Sour Sauce

These tasty meatballs in a sweet-and-sour sauce are a family favorite. Red meat provides the best source of iron for you and your child, since it is in a form that is absorbed well by the body. Lack of iron is the most common deficiency in children and will leave your child feeling tired and run-down and make him or her more prone to infection. It is useful to keep a stock of these meatballs in the freezer.

Makes 5 servings

1 pound lean ground beef
1 medium onion, finely chopped
1 apple, peeled and grated
½ cup fresh white bread crumbs
1 tablespoon chopped fresh parsley
1 chicken stock cube, finely crumbled
2 tablespoons cold water
Salt and freshly ground black pepper
2 tablespoons vegetable oil

Sweet-and-Sour Sauce
1 tablespoon soy sauce
1½ teaspoons cornstarch
1 tablespoon vegetable oil
1 medium onion, finely chopped
½ cup chopped sweet red pepper
One 14-ounce can of chopped tomatoes
1 tablespoon malt vinegar
1 teaspoon brown sugar
Freshly ground black pepper

Mix together all the ingredients for the meatballs except the vegetable oil and chop for a few seconds in a food processor. Using floured hands, form into about 20 meatballs. Heat the oil in a frying pan and sauté the meatballs for 10 to 12 minutes, turning occasionally, until browned.

Meanwhile, to make the sauce, mix together the soy sauce and cornstarch in a small bowl. Heat the oil in a pan and sauté the onion for 3 minutes. Add the red pepper and sauté, stirring occasionally, for 2 minutes. Add the tomatoes, vinegar, and sugar, season with black pepper, and simmer for 10 minutes. Add the soy sauce mixture and cook for 2 minutes, stirring occasionally. Blend and puree the sauce.

Pour the sauce over the meatballs, cover, and simmer for about 5 minutes or until cooked through.

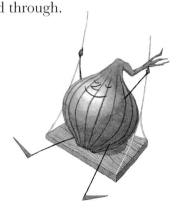

Mini Burgers with Cheese Stars

The apple in these burgers gives them a deliciously sweet taste and keeps them lovely and moist, too. Serve the burgers without the bun if you prefer.

Makes 12 small burgers

1 pound ground beef or lamb
1 medium onion, finely chopped
1 chicken stock cube, dissolved in
2 tablespoons boiling water
1 large apple, peeled and grated (squeeze out excess juice)
1 tablespoon chopped fresh parsley

Salt and freshly ground black pepper
Vegetable oil

Assorted mini rolls
Lettuce
Cheese slices, cut into stars
Tomato relish or ketchup

Mix together all the ingredients for the burgers except the vegetable oil and form into about 12 small burgers. Panfry in oil, broil, or barbecue the burgers. Cut the mini rolls in half and place the burgers on some lettuce and top with a cheese star. Leave out the cheese if you prefer and add some tomato relish or ketchup.

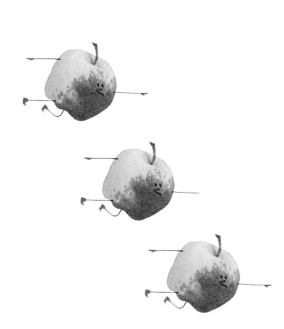

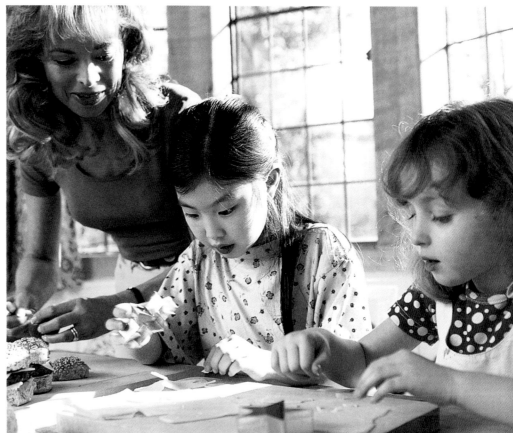

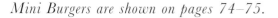

Mini Burgers are shown on pages 74–75.

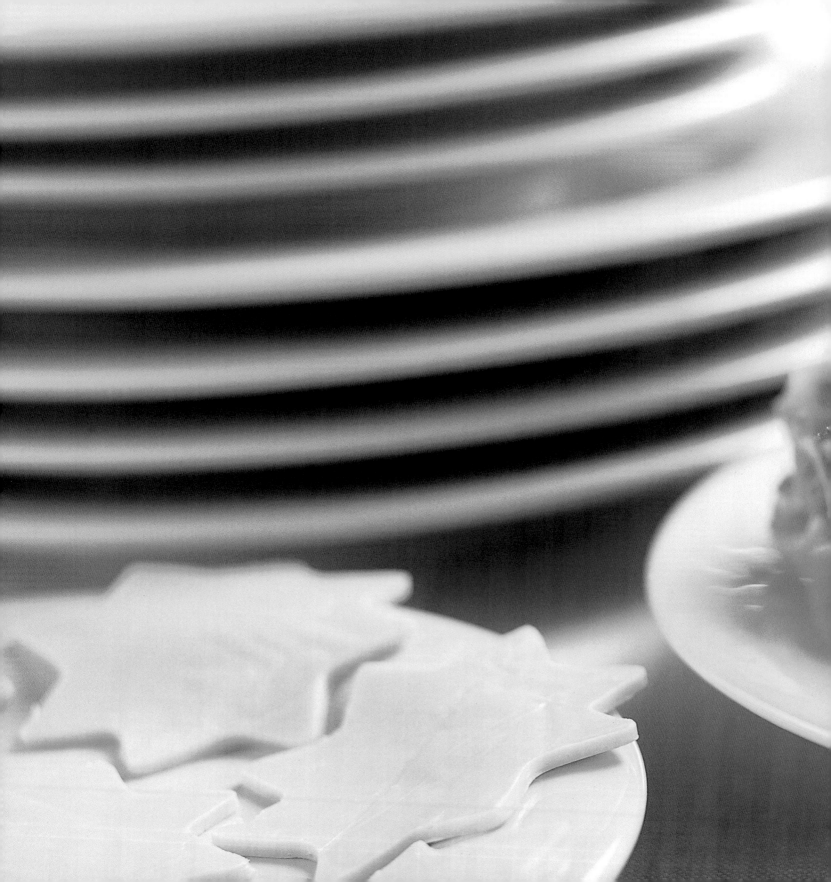

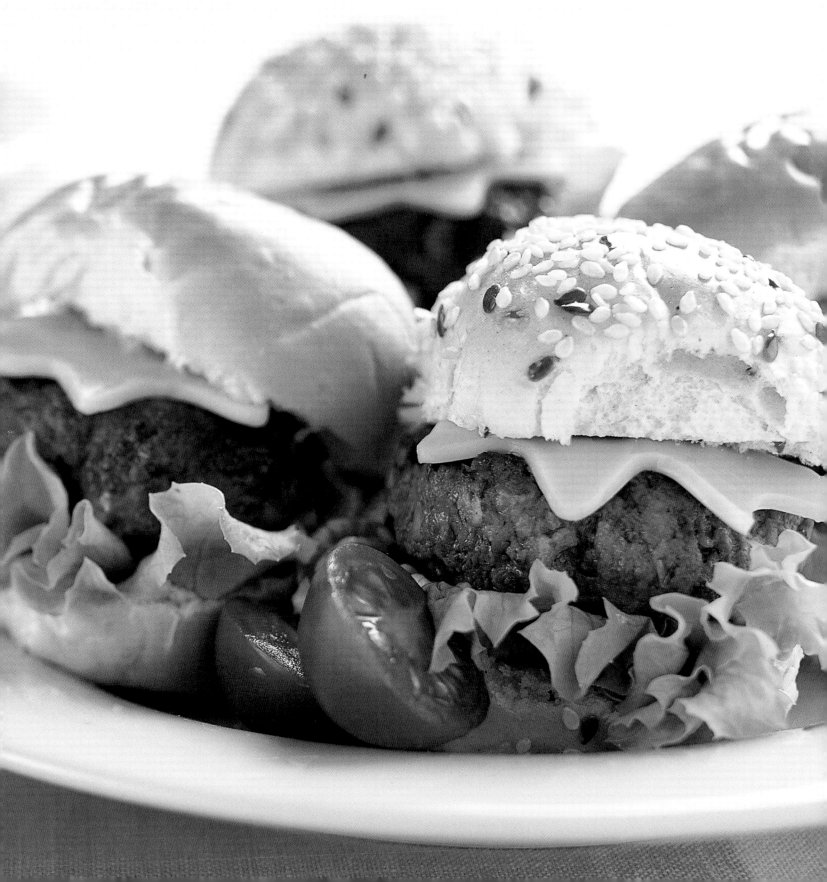

Honeyed Lamb Cutlets

Children like eating food with their fingers, which is one reason why lamb cutlets are popular. They are especially delicious if marinated in soy sauce and honey first.

Makes 6 lamb cutlets

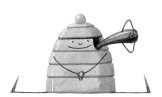

Marinade
2 tablespoons soy sauce
1 tablespoon honey
½ teaspoon sesame oil

6 lamb cutlets

Combine the ingredients for the marinade and marinate the cutlets for at least 2 hours or overnight. Cook under a preheated broiler for about 8 minutes, turning halfway through. Brush with the marinade during cooking.

Tasty Chinese-Style Chopped Beef

A lovely combination of tasty beef with crunchy water chestnuts. Serve on its own or with rice or noodles. This also makes a delicious filling for tortilla wraps or tacos.

Makes 4 servings

1 tablespoon sesame oil
½ small sweet red pepper
1 cup (1 or 2 small) finely chopped zucchini
1 medium onion, chopped
12 ounces ground beef
One 5-ounce can of water chestnuts,
drained and finely chopped

6 canned whole baby corn
1 cup bean sprouts
2 tablespoons oyster sauce
3 tablespoons rice wine vinegar

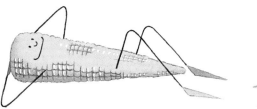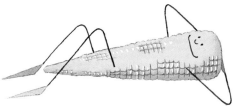

Heat the sesame oil in a wok or frying pan, add the red pepper, zucchini, and onion, and cook for 3 minutes. Meanwhile, fry the ground beef in a dry frying pan, stirring to break up with a fork until browned. Add the meat to the wok, stir in the water chestnuts, corn, and bean sprouts, and cook for 2 to 3 minutes. Stir in the oyster sauce and rice wine vinegar and stir-fry for 2 to 3 minutes, until slightly thickened.

Mexican Beef Tortillas

Tortillas are very popular with children, and this is delicious and simple to prepare.

Makes 6 tortillas

Marinade
1 teaspoon honey
1 tablespoon lime juice
Grated zest of half a lime
1 tablespoon soy sauce
1 large shallot, finely chopped
1 clove garlic, crushed
2 tablespoons olive oil

Vegetable oil for frying
8 ounces round steak or rump steak
1 ripe avocado
1½ tablespoons lemon juice
6 tortilla wraps
Handful of shredded lettuce
¼ cup sour cream

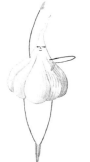

Mix the ingredients for the marinade together, and marinate the steak for at least 2 hours, turning occasionally to infuse the flavors.

Heat a dash of oil in a griddle pan until smoking, then add the steak and cook for about 3 minutes on each side, depending on the thickness of the steak. Remove from the pan and leave to rest for a few minutes before cutting into thin slices. If you don't have a griddle pan, you can use a frying pan.

Halve, pit, peel, and slice the avocado and toss quickly in the lemon juice. Heat the tortillas for a few seconds in the microwave (this makes them more pliable). Arrange some shredded lettuce in the center of each tortilla and cover with the sliced avocado, beef strips, and about 2 teaspoons of sour cream. Fold over the bottom of the tortilla, then fold in the sides and press to seal.

Marinated Beef with Vegetables

This delicious, quick, and easy to prepare beef stir-fry is bound to become a family favorite.
It makes a great all-in-one meal.

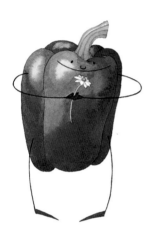

Makes 4 or 5 servings

Marinade
1 tablespoon soy sauce
1 tablespoon sake or sherry
1 teaspoon sesame oil
1 teaspoon cornstarch

8 ounces round steak, rump steak, or sirloin,
cut into strips
8 ounces pasta twirls
1 medium carrot, peeled and sliced
or cut into stars
6 ounces new potatoes
4 ounces green beans, trimmed

3 tablespoons sunflower oil
1 clove garlic, crushed
1 medium onion, thinly sliced

Sauce
½ chicken stock cube, dissolved in
6 tablespoons boiling water
½ teaspoon rice wine vinegar
1 teaspoon soy sauce
1 teaspoon sugar
½ teaspoon cornstarch

½ sweet red pepper, cut into strips
Salt and freshly ground black pepper

TIP
You can marinate foods in plastic bags instead of bowls that you have to wash up. Be sure you flip the bag from time to time to make sure everything gets a good soak.

Mix together the ingredients for the marinade and marinate the beef strips for at least 20 minutes. Cook the pasta in a large pot of lightly salted boiling water according to the instructions on the package, drain, set aside, and keep warm. Steam the carrot, potatoes, and green beans for about 6 minutes or until tender.

Meanwhile, heat 1 tablespoon of the oil in a wok or frying pan and stir-fry the beef for 3 minutes. Take out the beef and set aside. In the same pan, heat the remaining 2 tablespoons oil and sauté the garlic and onion for 3 minutes. Mix together all the ingredients for the sauce. Add the red pepper to the onion and cook for 2 minutes, cut the potatoes into slices, and add these together with the carrot, green beans, and beef and season with some salt and freshly ground black pepper. Stir in the sauce and cooked pasta and cook for 2 minutes.

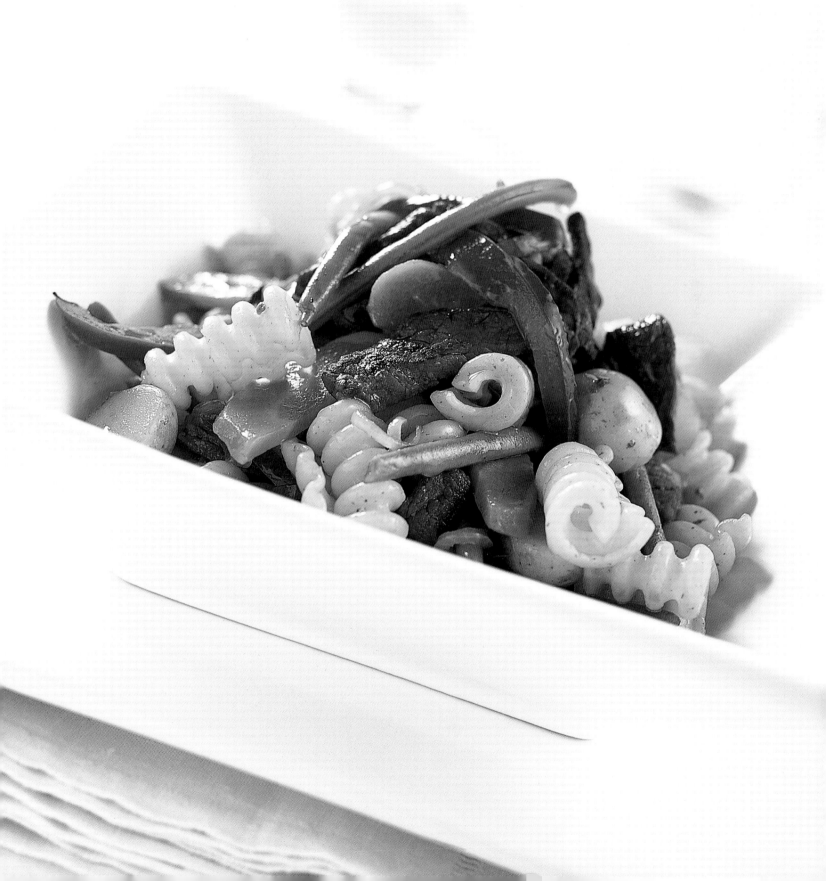

Marinated Beef Skewers

Marinating cubes of beef in this sauce gives them a delicious flavor and also tenderizes the meat. This is a particular favorite of my three children. If you prefer, you can make these skewers very successfully without the vegetables.

Makes 3 or 4 servings

Marinade
½-inch piece of gingerroot, peeled and grated
1 clove garlic, crushed
1 tablespoon dark soy sauce
1 teaspoon rice wine vinegar
1 tablespoon vegetable oil
1 tablespoon honey

12 ounces round steak, cut into cubes
½ sweet red pepper, cut into chunks
1 small onion, cut into chunks
4 button mushrooms
Vegetable oil

Mix together all the ingredients for the marinade and marinate the cubes of beef for at least 1 hour. Toss the red pepper, onion, and mushrooms in a little vegetable oil and thread onto the skewers alternately with the cubes of beef. Place on foil in a broiler pan and broil for 3 to 4 minutes on each side.

Beef Tacos

Tacos (crispy toasted corn shells) originated in Mexico and the word *taco* means "snack." You can buy taco kits containing shells, spice mix, and salsa in the supermarket. This beef mixture is also good wrapped in a tortilla.

Makes 6 tacos

1 tablespoon vegetable oil
1 small onion, finely chopped
1 clove garlic, crushed
8 ounces ground beef
2 tablespoons taco spice mix
6 taco shells

3 tablespoons salsa
Handful of shredded lettuce
2 chopped tomatoes
Grated Monterey Jack cheese
Guacamole or sour cream (optional)

Heat the vegetable oil in a pan and sauté the onion and garlic until softened, about 3 minutes. Add the ground beef and brown. Drain the excess liquid. Add the taco spice mix and 2 tablespoons water. Bring to a boil, then simmer for 10 minutes, stirring occasionally.

Heat the taco shells in the microwave. Fill with the ground beef, salsa, lettuce, tomatoes, and cheese. Top with guacamole or sour cream if you like.

Sesame Beef Stir-fry

This recipe is a firm family favorite in my house. I usually make it using round steak cut into thin strips (see photograph, page 70).

Makes 4 servings

1 tablespoon sesame oil
1 clove garlic, crushed
1 medium carrot, peeled and cut into matchsticks
8 canned whole baby corn, cut in half
1 zucchini, cut into matchsticks
10 ounces round steak or rump steak, cut into very fine strips

1 tablespoon cornstarch
½ cup beef stock
2 tablespoons dark brown sugar
2 tablespoons soy sauce
A few drops of Tabasco sauce
1 tablespoon sesame seeds

Heat the sesame oil in a wok and stir-fry the garlic, carrot, corn, and zucchini for 3 to 4 minutes. Add the beef strips and continue to stir-fry for 4 to 5 minutes. Mix the cornstarch together with 1 tablespoon of water and stir into the beef stock. Stir this into the wok together with the sugar, soy sauce, Tabasco, and sesame seeds. Bring to a simmer, cook until slightly thickened, and serve with rice.

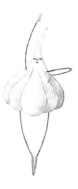

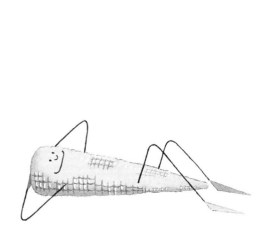

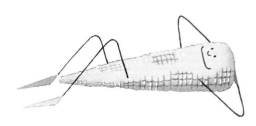

Simon's Multilayered Cottage Pie

Luckily, my husband, Simon, loves nursery food. His all-time favorite meal would probably be cottage pie followed by gelatin. So, especially for him, I have concocted this rather luxurious version of a perennial family favorite. For adults you can increase the amount of Worcestershire sauce to give this a more tangy flavor.

Makes 5 servings

1 tablespoon vegetable oil
1 large onion, finely chopped
1 pound ground beef or lamb
One 14-ounce can of chopped tomatoes
1 cup chicken or beef stock
1 teaspoon mixed herbs
2 teaspoons Worcestershire sauce
1 tablespoon tomato sauce
Salt and freshly ground black pepper

1 pound carrots, peeled and sliced
1 teaspoon plus 4 tablespoons butter
1¼ pounds potatoes, peeled and chopped

5 tablespoons milk
Salt and freshly ground black pepper
1 medium onion, finely chopped
1½ teaspoons vegetable oil
1½ cups frozen peas
1 cup chicken stock

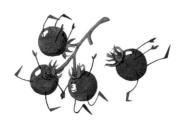

Preheat the oven to 350°F. Heat the oil in a frying pan and sauté the onion until softened. Stir in the meat and cook until well browned, stirring occasionally. Add the tomatoes, stock, herbs, Worcestershire sauce, tomato sauce, and seasoning. Bring to a boil, then reduce the heat and cover and simmer for 30 minutes.

Meanwhile, cook the carrots until quite soft, then mash with the 1 teaspoon butter until smooth. At the same time, cook the potatoes in boiling salted water until tender. Drain and mash them with the 4 tablespoons butter and the milk, and season to taste. Sauté the onion in the vegetable oil until softened, stir in the peas, and pour the stock over the top. Bring to a boil and then simmer for 3 minutes.

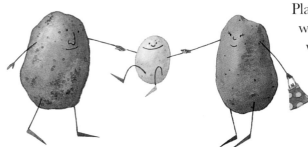

Place the meat in an ovenproof glass dish, top with the peas, then cover with the carrots and finally with a layer of mashed potatoes. Dot the top with a little butter and bake in the oven for about 20 minutes. Finish off for a few minutes under a preheated broiler to brown the topping.

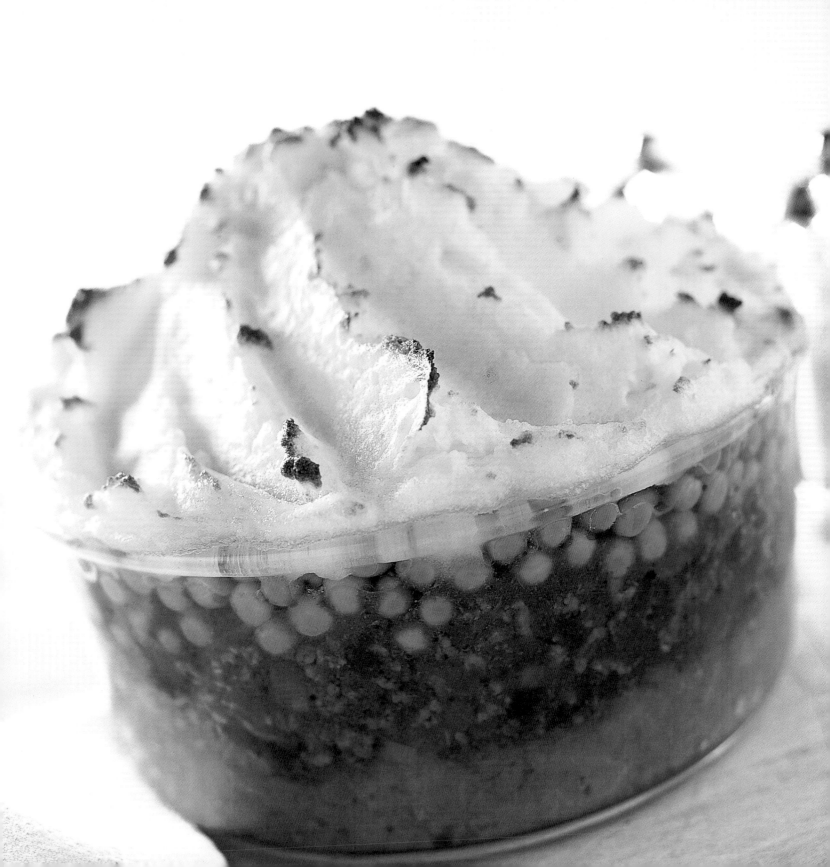

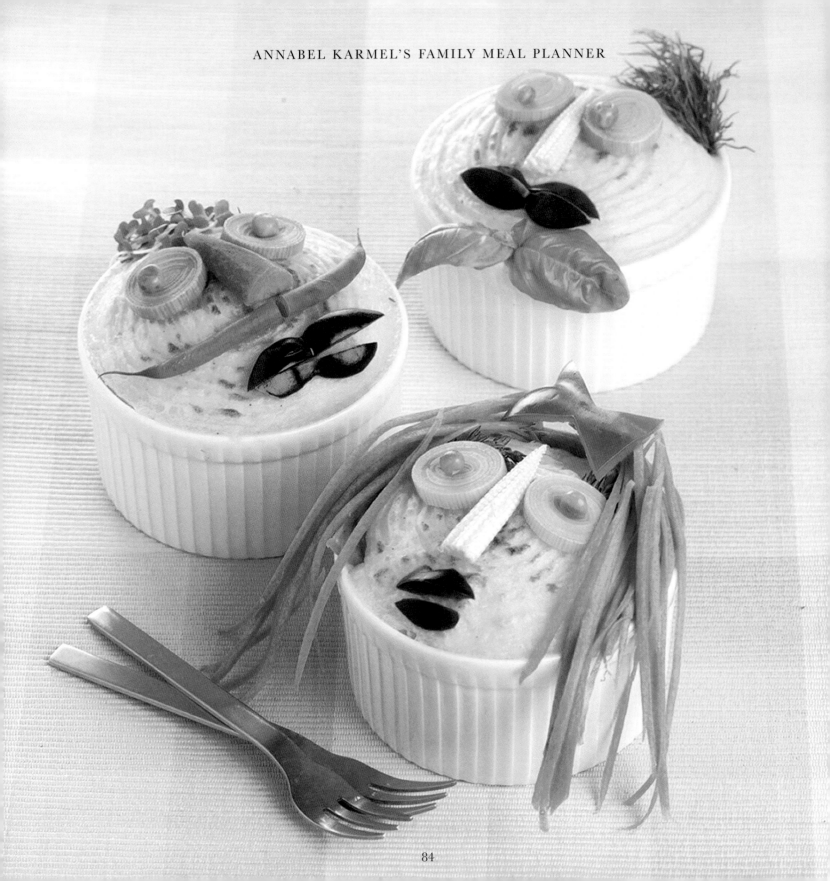

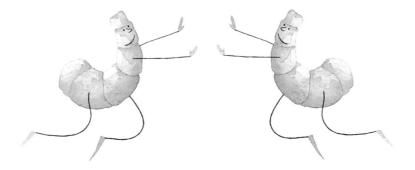

Fish

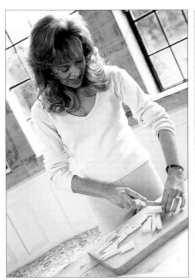
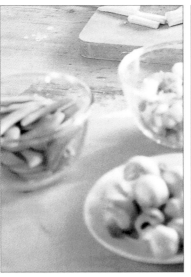
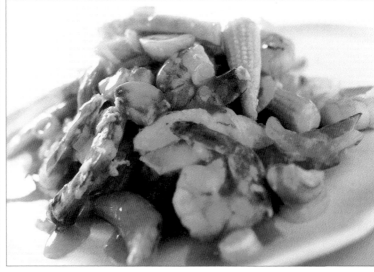

Very Easy Florentine Fillets

Fillets of tender white fish on a bed of fresh spinach covered with cheese sauce is a classic and favorite combination.

**Makes 2
servings**

8 ounces fresh spinach or
4 ounces frozen spinach
2 tablespoons butter, plus extra
for dotting the fish
Salt and freshly ground black pepper

½ cup heavy cream
¼ cup grated Parmesan cheese
8 ounces fillet of cod or haddock, skinned
1 tablespoon milk
¼ cup grated Swiss or Cheddar cheese

Wash the spinach and remove any tough stalks. Cook in a saucepan with just a little water clinging to the leaves, until wilted. Squeeze out any excess moisture. Melt 1 tablespoon of the butter and sauté the spinach for 1 minute and season to taste. (Alternatively, the spinach can be cooked in a microwave.)

Meanwhile, put the cream, the remaining 1 tablespoon butter, and the Parmesan cheese in a small saucepan and heat gently until the butter has melted. Lightly season the fish, put into a suitable container, dot with butter, and pour over the milk. Cook in a microwave on high for about 4 minutes or until the fish flakes easily with a fork. (Alternatively, the fish can be cooked under a preheated broiler.)

Pour the cooking liquid from the fish into the cheese sauce. Arrange the spinach on a greased ovenproof dish and place the fish fillets on top. Pour over the cheese sauce and sprinkle with the grated Swiss or Cheddar cheese. Brown under a preheated broiler for 2 to 3 minutes.

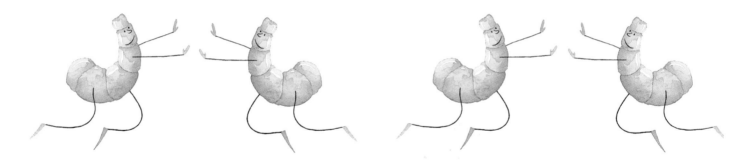

Tasty 10-Minute Shrimp Stir-fry

Here is a tasty stir-fry with colorful crunchy vegetables and carrot curls that is very quick to prepare.
It is good served with Perfect Chinese Fried Rice (page 116).

**Makes 4
servings**

8 canned whole baby corn
1 medium carrot, peeled
1½ teaspoons vegetable oil
2 scallions, sliced
4 ounces sugar snap peas
1 cup chicken stock

1 tablespoon soy sauce
2 tablespoons sake or sherry
2 tablespoons cornstarch
8 ounces cooked shrimp

Halve the corn lengthwise, then cut across in half again. Using a potato peeler, cut thin strips from the carrot, and cut these in half again to make long, thin, curly strips. Heat the oil in a wok or frying pan and sauté the scallions for 1 minute. Add the other vegetables and stir-fry for 2 to 3 minutes. Remove the vegetables and set aside. Mix together the chicken stock, soy sauce, sake or sherry, and cornstarch. Pour the mixture into the wok and stir constantly while bringing to a boil. Reduce the heat and simmer, stirring, for 1 to 2 minutes, until thickened. Stir in the shrimp and the vegetables and heat through.

Teriyaki-Glazed Trout Fillets

Oily fish such as salmon, trout, tuna, and mackerel contain omega-3 fatty acids that help to reduce the risk of heart disease and strokes, as well as being important for brain development.

**Makes 2
servings**

Marinade
2 tablespoons soy sauce
2 tablespoons sake or sherry
2 tablespoons mirin

4 trout fillets

Mix together all the ingredients for the marinade in a small saucepan and bring to a boil. Simmer for 2 to 3 minutes. Arrange the trout fillets in a shallow dish and pour over the hot marinade. Set aside for about 15 minutes. Preheat the broiler and lay the fillets on a broiler pan lined with foil and broil for 5 to 6 minutes on the fleshy side, until cooked. Pour the sauce over the fillets.

Shrimp Stir-fry with Sugar Snap Peas

Stir-fries make popular, quick, and easy meals for the whole family, especially if you have a quantity of chicken stock prepared ahead and in the freezer. This particular recipe can also be made with fresh uncooked shrimp.

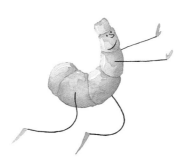

Makes 4 servings

Marinade
1 egg white, lightly beaten
1 teaspoon cornstarch
Pinch of salt
Pinch of ground white pepper

10 ounces cooked shrimp

Sauce
1½ cups chicken stock
1 tablespoon soy sauce
1 tablespoon sesame oil
1½ tablespoons superfine sugar

1½ teaspoons cider vinegar
1½ tablespoons cornstarch
2 scallions, finely sliced
Ground white pepper

3 tablespoons vegetable oil
2 eggs, lightly beaten
1 clove garlic, crushed
1 medium onion, thinly sliced
8 canned whole baby corn, cut in half
1 cup halved button mushrooms
5 ounces sugar snap peas

Mix together the beaten egg white, cornstarch, and seasoning and marinate the shrimp in this mixture for about 10 minutes. To make the sauce, mix together the stock, soy sauce, sesame oil, sugar, and vinegar. In a small bowl mix 3 tablespoons of the sauce with the cornstarch until smooth and then stir this into the rest of the sauce. Pour the sauce into a saucepan, bring to a boil, and then simmer, stirring, for 2 to 3 minutes, until thickened. Stir in the scallions and season with a little white pepper.

Strain the marinade from the shrimp and discard. Heat 1 tablespoon of the oil in a frying pan and sauté the shrimp for about 2 minutes, then set aside. Heat another tablespoon of oil in the pan and swirl the beaten eggs around to form a thin layer, and cook until set. Remove from the pan and fold it over three times like a Swiss roll, cut into strips, and set aside.

Add the remaining 1 tablespoon oil to the pan and sauté the garlic and onion for 2 minutes. Stir-fry the corn, button mushrooms, and sugar snap peas for 6 minutes. Add the shrimp, egg strips, and the sauce and cook for 2 minutes or until heated through.

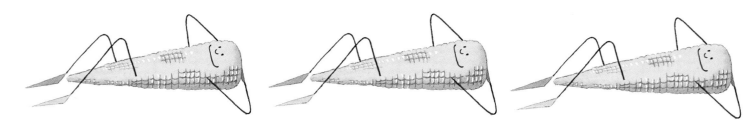

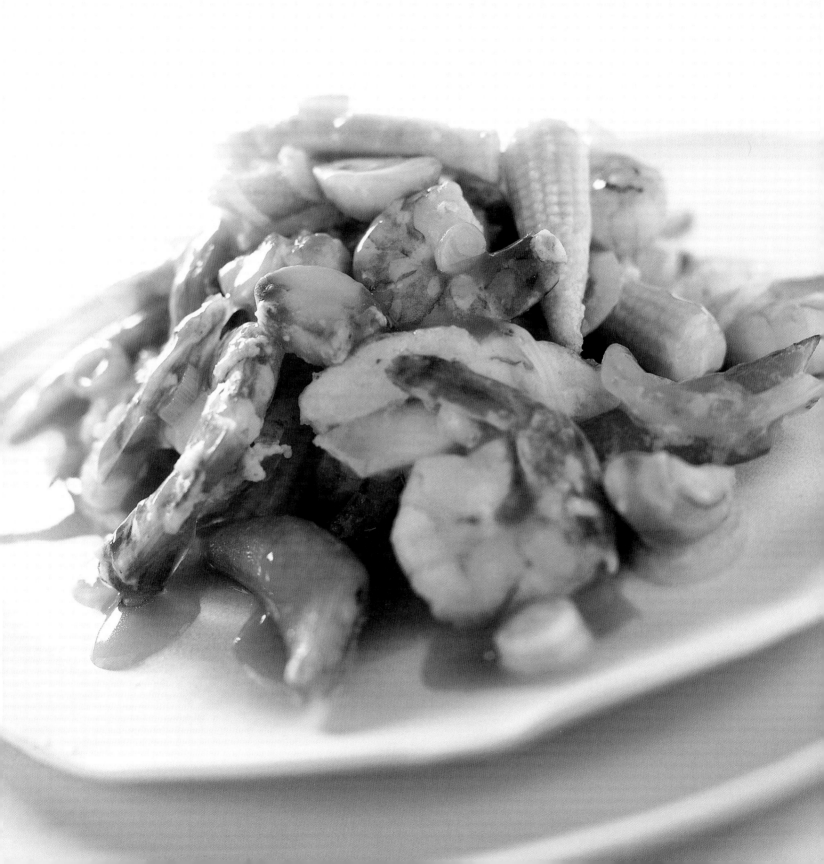

Yummy Fish in Orange Sauce

This is a great way to cook up a fillet of fresh fish in just a few minutes. Since it is so easy, I make it for my own lunch sometimes. For more servings, simply increase the quantities.

Makes 1 serving

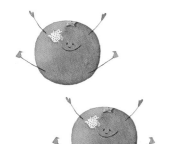

All-purpose flour
Salt and freshly ground black pepper
8 ounces fillet of cod, haddock,
or hake, skinned

1 tablespoon butter
1 teaspoon soy sauce
1 teaspoon freshly squeezed orange juice

Season some flour with a little salt and freshly ground black pepper and coat the fish in the seasoned flour. Melt the butter in a frying pan and sauté the fish for about 5 minutes, turning occasionally. Mix together the soy sauce and orange juice, pour over the fish, turn up the heat, and cook for about 1 minute.

Mermaid Morsels

These miniature fish balls are very tasty. You can use any combination of white fish available, such as cod, haddock, whiting, hake, or halibut. A fishmonger should be able to prepare it for you. They are good served hot or cold.

Makes 20 balls

1 large onion, finely chopped
1 tablespoon vegetable oil, plus extra
for frying the fish balls
1 teaspoon butter, plus extra
for frying the fish balls
1 pound finely chopped white fish
1 carrot, peeled and finely grated

1 tablespoon finely chopped fresh parsley
1 egg, lightly beaten
2 teaspoons sugar
1 teaspoon salt
Freshly ground black pepper
2 tablespoons all-purpose flour, plus extra
for coating the fish balls

Fry the onion in a mixture of the oil and butter until soft and lightly golden. Combine the chopped fish, fried onion, carrot, and parsley. Beat the egg together with the sugar, salt, and a little pepper until frothy and add the egg mixture to the fish. Finally, mix in 1½ tablespoons cold water and the 2 tablespoons flour. Using your hands, form into small walnut-size balls, roll in flour, and fry in a mixture of vegetable oil and butter until golden, turning occasionally.

Spaghetti Marinara

It is very important that you buy only very fresh seafood, so always buy it from a reputable source. This is a delicious pasta sauce, and you can make it quite spicy for adults by adding more chile if you like. I would not recommend giving seafood to very young children.

**Makes 4
servings**

2 pounds mussels
8 large raw shrimp
12 ounces spaghetti

Sauce
2 tablespoons olive oil
4 shallots, finely chopped

1 clove garlic, crushed
2 tablespoons chopped fresh parsley
6 tablespoons dry white wine
One 28½-ounce can of chopped tomatoes
1 or 2 dried red chiles, crushed, or a good
pinch of red pepper flakes
Salt and freshly ground black pepper

Discard any mussels that are not closed, then scrub well under cold water and pull off and discard the beards. Set the mussels aside. Peel, devein, and cut the shrimp in half lengthwise. Cook the spaghetti in a large pot of lightly salted boiling water according to the instructions on the package.

Heat the olive oil in a frying pan and sauté the shallots and garlic for 2 minutes; add the parsley and sauté for 1 minute. Add the wine, simmer for 2 minutes, then add the tomatoes and chile and simmer for 4 minutes. Add the mussels and cook for 4 to 5 minutes. Discard any mussels that do not open. Add the shrimp, simmer for about 2 minutes, and season to taste.

Drain the spaghetti, return to the warm pot, add the marinara sauce, and toss gently. If you like, remove the mussels from their shells and mix with the spaghetti.

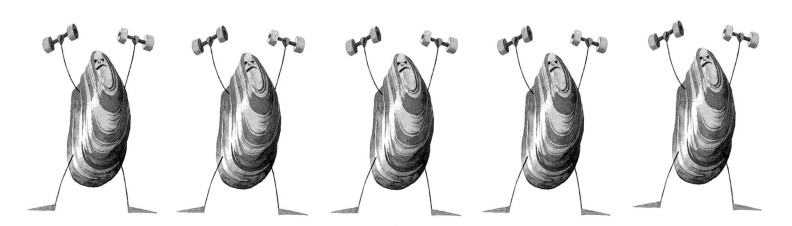

Simply Super Salmon Teriyaki

Oily fish such as salmon, trout, tuna, and mackerel contain omega-3 fatty acids, which protect against heart disease and strokes. The old wives' tale that fish is good for the brain is true, since omega-3 essential fats optimize messaging between nerve cells in the brain. This is vital for proper brain functioning, and research suggests that a diet rich in omega-3 fats can also improve the performance of children who suffer from attention deficit disorder.

My children and I all love Japanese food, and it is well worth investing in bottles of sake and mirin (a sweet Japanese cooking wine), as you will want to make this recipe over and over again. Serve with basmati rice.

Makes 4 servings

Marinade
6 tablespoons soy sauce
½ cup sake (rice wine)
¼ cup mirin (sweet sake for cooking)
2 tablespoons sugar

4 thick salmon fillets (approximately 5 ounces each), skinned
2 tablespoons vegetable oil
1 cup sliced button mushrooms
1 cup bean sprouts

Mix the ingredients for the marinade together in a saucepan and stir over medium heat until the sugar has dissolved. Marinate the salmon in the sauce for 10 minutes.

Heat 1 tablespoon of the oil and sauté the mushrooms for 2 minutes, then add the bean sprouts and cook for 2 minutes more. Meanwhile, drain the salmon, reserving the marinade. Heat the remaining 1 tablespoon oil in a frying pan and sauté the salmon for 1 to 2 minutes on each side or until slightly browned. Pour away the excess oil from the frying pan. Alternatively, it is particularly good if you cook the salmon on a very hot griddle pan brushed with a little oil.

Whichever method you choose, after 2 minutes pour a little of the teriyaki marinade over the salmon and continue to cook for a few minutes, basting occasionally. Simmer the remaining marinade in a small saucepan until thickened. Divide the vegetables among four plates, place the salmon on top, and pour the teriyaki sauce over the fish.

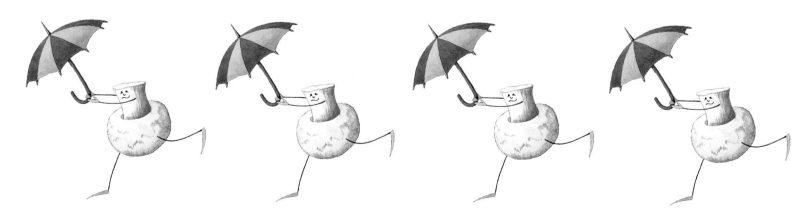

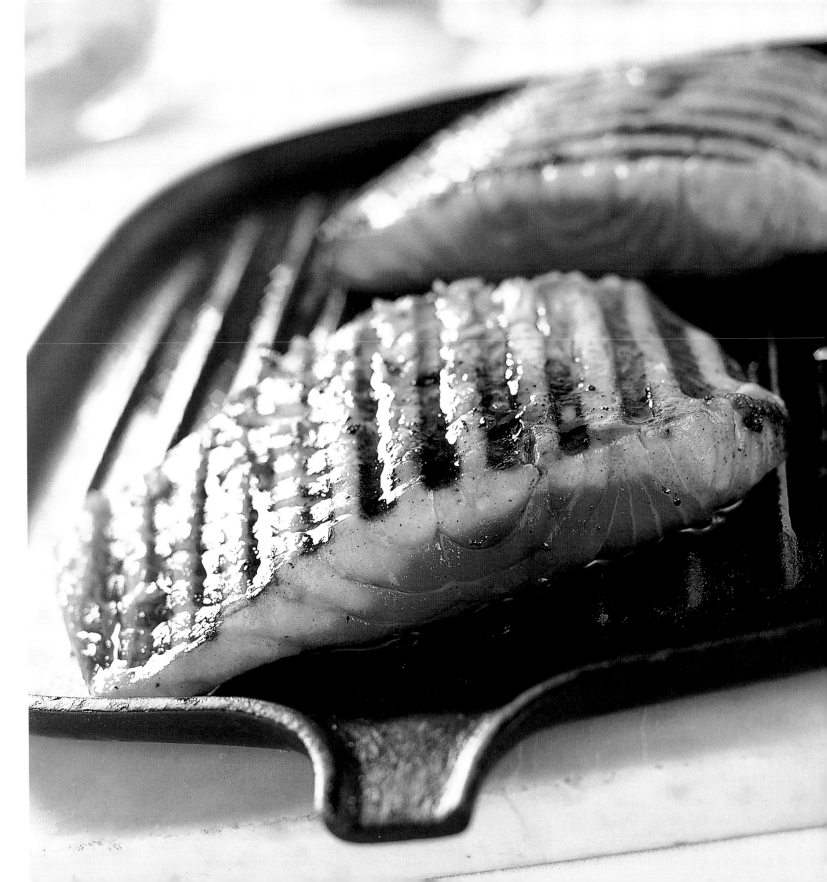

Fishing for Compliments

It's a shame that for many children the only fish that they enjoy eating is fish sticks. However, this is a very tasty fish recipe that I have invented for children, although it's also delicious for the whole family and may well tempt even the most reluctant fish eater.

Makes 2 servings

12 ounces flounder, sole, or cod fillets, skinned and cut into strips 2½ inches long
1 tablespoon lemon juice
1 tablespoon chopped onion

Sauce
1 cup chicken stock
2 teaspoons soy sauce
1 teaspoon sesame oil
1 tablespoon sugar

1 teaspoon cider vinegar
1 tablespoon cornstarch
1 scallion, finely sliced

3 tablespoons vegetable oil
2 small zucchini, cut into strips
½ sweet red pepper, cut into strips
All-purpose flour
Salt and freshly ground black pepper

Rinse the fish fillets and pat dry with paper towels. Mix together the lemon juice and chopped onion with 1 tablespoon water and marinate the fish in this mixture for about 30 minutes.

To make the sauce, mix together the stock, soy sauce, sesame oil, sugar, vinegar, and cornstarch. Pour the sauce into a saucepan, bring to a boil, and then simmer, stirring, for 2 to 3 minutes, until thickened and smooth. Stir in the scallion.

Heat 1 tablespoon of the vegetable oil in a pan and sauté the zucchini and red pepper for 4 minutes. Strain the marinade from the fish and discard (including the onion), then coat the fish lightly in seasoned flour. Heat the remaining 2 tablespoons oil in a pan and sauté the fish for about 3 minutes on each side or until cooked. Add the vegetables, pour over the sauce, and cook for 2 minutes.

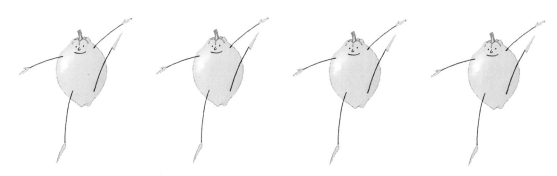

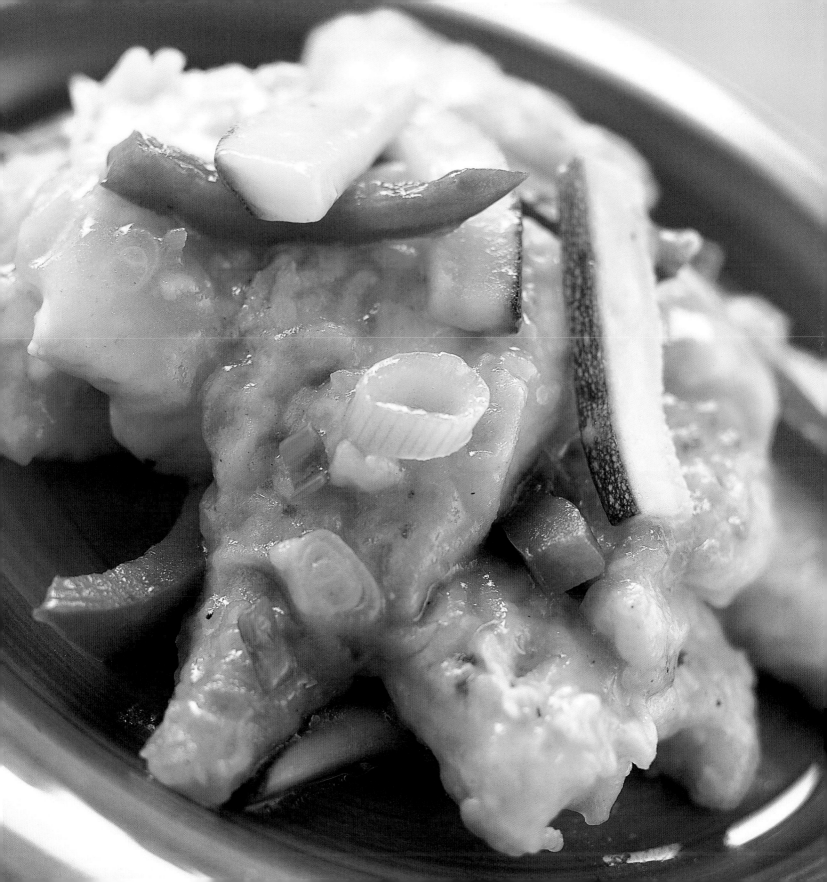

Individual New England Fish Pies

If you want your child to grow up liking fish, then you should try these delicious mini fish pies. It is nice to make individual portions for your child in ramekin dishes—much more appealing than a dollop of fish pie on a plate. You can store extra portions in the freezer for days when you don't want to cook. Before serving you can decorate them with faces made from vegetables and herbs if you like (see photograph, page 84).

Makes 4 mini fish pies

2 pounds potatoes, peeled and chopped
8 ounces haddock, cod, scrod, or whitefish fillets, skinned and cut into chunks
2 cups plus ¼ cup milk
6 peppercorns
1 bay leaf
1 parsley sprig
7 tablespoons butter
6 ounces scallops

6 ounces shrimp, peeled and deveined
(or use 12 ounces scallops or shrimp)
1 medium onion, finely chopped
3 tablespoons all-purpose flour
½ cup grated Cheddar cheese
Salt and freshly ground white pepper
½ cup frozen peas
1 egg, lightly beaten

For the mashed potatoes, boil some lightly salted water, add the potatoes, and boil until tender.

Meanwhile, put the fish into a shallow pan with the 2 cups milk, the peppercorns, and herbs. Bring to a boil, then reduce the heat, cover, and simmer for 5 minutes or until the fish flakes easily. Remove the fish, strain the milk, and reserve. Flake the fish with a fork, checking carefully for bones, and set aside.

Melt 2 tablespoons of the butter in a pan and sauté the scallops and shrimp for 2 minutes, remove with a slotted spoon, and then cut in half.

Melt 4 tablespoons of the butter in a saucepan, add the onion, and sauté until softened. Stir in the flour to make a paste and cook for 1 minute. Gradually add the strained milk, stirring until the sauce thickens. Remove from the heat and stir in the grated cheese until melted. Season to taste, then stir in the frozen peas, the fish, and the shrimp and scallops. Spoon the mixture into 4 ramekin dishes.

Drain and mash the potatoes. Add the remaining 1 tablespoon butter, the ¼ cup milk, and salt and freshly ground white pepper. Spread the potatoes over the fish mixture in the ramekin dishes, making lines on the surface using a fork. Brush with the beaten egg.

Place in a preheated 375°F oven for 15 to 20 minutes, and finish off under a preheated broiler until browned. Decorate with faces if you like.

Posh Fish Fingers

Crushed cornflakes make a delicious coating for fried fish. Serve with low-fat oven fries and maybe wrap them up in a newspaper or a comic for fun. My children like fish and chips sprinkled with a little malt vinegar.

**Makes 4
servings**

¼ cup cornflakes
1 tablespoon chopped fresh parsley
1 pound cod, haddock, or hake fillets, skinned
Salt and freshly ground black pepper

½ cup all-purpose flour
1 egg, lightly beaten
Vegetable oil

Crush the cornflakes (this can be done by putting them in a bag and crushing them with a rolling pin) and mix with the chopped parsley. Divide the fish into 4 portions and season. Coat in the flour and then dip into the beaten egg. Roll the fish fillets into the cornflake mixture to coat and fry in vegetable oil until golden and cooked through.

Perfect Paella

This paella is simple and quick to prepare. It is very important that you use only fresh live mussels, and any uncooked mussels that are already open should be discarded. Once the mussels are cooked the shells should open, but do not eat cooked mussels if the shells remain closed. You can sometimes buy bags of frozen or fresh mixed seafood, which can also be used for this recipe, and then you may find that the mussels are already cooked and out of their shells (see photograph, pages 98–99).

**Makes 4
servings**

1 medium onion, chopped
1 clove garlic, crushed
1 tablespoon olive oil
1 sweet red pepper, cut into strips
1¼ cups rice
1 teaspoon ground turmeric
1 teaspoon mild chili powder

4 cups chicken stock
1 bay leaf
2 tablespoons chopped fresh parsley
5 ounces shrimp, peeled and deveined
8 ounces clams
12 ounces mussels
1 cup frozen peas

Sauté the onion and garlic in the oil for 1 minute. Add the red pepper and cook for another 3 minutes. Add the rice and the turmeric and chili powder and stir in the pan for about 1 minute. Pour in the stock, add the bay leaf, and cook for 15 minutes over medium heat. Add the parsley and cook for about 5 minutes. Turn the heat up, add the seafood and frozen peas, and cook for 1 to 2 minutes over high heat. Reduce the heat, cover, and cook for about 5 minutes or until the seafood is cooked. Remove any mussels and clams that have not opened.

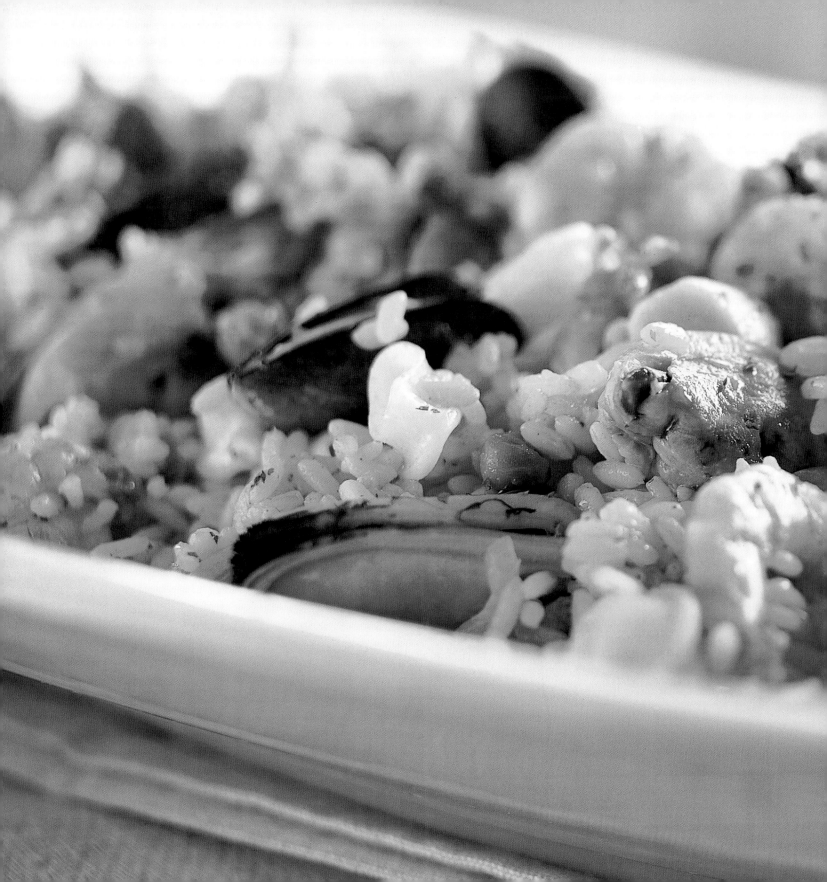

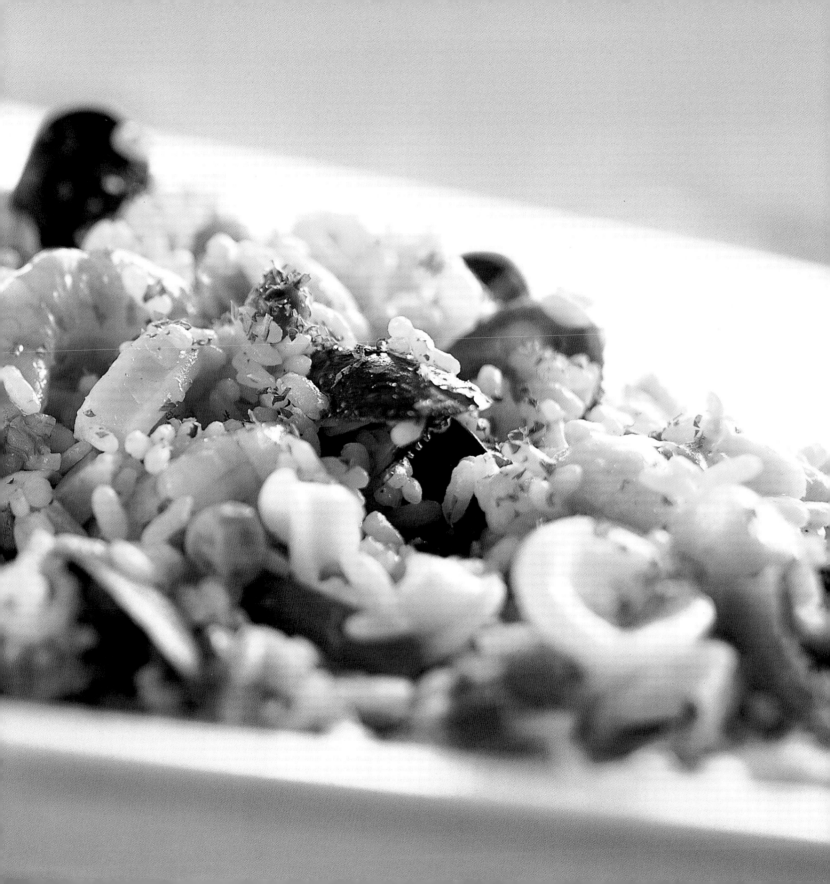

Maryland Crab Cakes

This is a very versatile recipe that will please both children and adults. You can make small cakes for perfect hors d'oeuvres or large cakes for an entrée or even a sandwich. The secret is to add only as much bread crumbs as needed to hold the patties together.

Makes 4 or 5 servings

12 ounces crabmeat, carefully picked over for shell
1 teaspoon prepared mustard, preferably Dijon
2 teaspoons Old Bay seasoning
2 tablespoons finely diced sweet red pepper
1 large egg, lightly beaten
2 tablespoons mayonnaise

Salt and freshly ground black pepper
½ cup bread crumbs
2 tablespoons butter or olive oil

Mix the crabmeat, mustard, Old Bay, red pepper, egg, mayonnaise, and salt and pepper. Add 2 tablespoons of the bread crumbs and try forming one-quarter of the mixture into a patty. If it does not hold together well, add another tablespoon of the bread crumbs, 1 teaspoon at a time, until the mixture holds together.

Pour the remaining 6 tablespoons bread crumbs onto a plate and carefully coat the patties.

Heat the butter or olive oil over medium-high heat in a nonstick skillet. Add the patties and cook until golden brown, about 4 minutes. Carefully flip and continue cooking for another 2 to 3 minutes.

Remove to a plate and serve with coleslaw, or as a sandwich with lettuce and tomato.

Optional ingredient: ¼ cup fresh corn, in which case you may need a tablespoon of flour and some additional mayonnaise to hold the patties together.

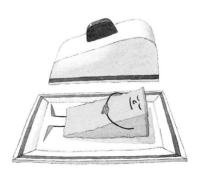

Soupa Tuna Tagliatelle

This is a tasty and nutritious pasta dish that is quick and easy to make for the whole family using cupboard ingredients, including a can of tomato soup.

Makes 6 servings

8 ounces green and white tagliatelle
2 tablespoons butter
1 small onion, finely chopped
1 heaping tablespoon cornstarch
One 10¾-ounce can of cream
of tomato soup
2 tablespoons chopped fresh parsley
½ teaspoon dried mixed herbs
Two 6-ounce cans of tuna in oil, drained

Cheese Sauce
2 tablespoons butter
1½ teaspoons all-purpose flour

1½ cups milk
Pinch of ground mustard
¾ cup grated Cheddar cheese
1 tablespoon snipped fresh chives
½ cup cooked corn kernels
Salt and freshly ground black pepper

Topping
2 tablespoons bread crumbs
¼ cup grated Cheddar cheese
1 tablespoon grated Parmesan cheese

Preheat the oven to 350°F. Cook the tagliatelle in a large pot of lightly salted boiling water until just tender. Melt the butter in a saucepan and sauté the onion until softened. Mix the cornstarch with 2 tablespoons of cold water until dissolved. Mix the cornstarch mixture, tomato soup, parsley, and herbs with the sautéed onion and cook over medium heat for about 5 minutes or until the sauce has thickened. Stir the tuna fish into the sauce and mix with the drained tagliatelle.

To make the cheese sauce, put the butter, flour, and milk into a saucepan and cook over medium heat. Using a balloon whisk, keep whisking the mixture until it boils and thickens to form a smooth sauce. Add the ground mustard and simmer for 2 to 3 minutes. Remove from the heat and stir in the cheese until melted. Stir in the chives and cooked corn and season to taste.

Arrange the tuna and pasta mixture in a 9-inch square ovenproof dish and pour over the cheese sauce. Mix together the bread crumbs and grated cheeses and scatter over the top. Bake in the oven for 20 minutes. Brown under a preheated broiler for a few minutes before serving.

Chinese Noodles with Shrimp and Bean Sprouts

This noodle dish is quick and easy to prepare and very versatile. You can use shredded chicken or pork instead of the shrimp or perhaps strips of omelet if you are vegetarian. You can also substitute other vegetables such as strips of zucchini, carrot, or baby sweet corn. This makes a good accompaniment to stir-fries.

Makes 4 servings

8 ounces medium egg noodles
2 tablespoons vegetable oil
4 scallions, sliced
½ to 1 teaspoon finely chopped red chile (optional)
1 clove garlic, crushed
1 tablespoon chopped fresh parsley
1 cup sliced button, oyster, or shiitake mushrooms

4 ounces peeled cooked large shrimp
3 tablespoons oyster sauce
1 teaspoon superfine sugar
½ cup water
1 cup bean sprouts
½ cup chicken stock

Drop the noodles into a large pot of boiling water. Return to a boil and simmer for 4 minutes. Drain and set aside.

Meanwhile, heat the vegetable oil in a wok or frying pan and stir-fry the scallions, chile, if using, garlic, and parsley for 1 minute. Add the mushrooms and shrimp and stir-fry for 2 minutes. Add the oyster sauce, sugar, and water. Stir in the bean sprouts and stock and cook for 2 minutes. Add the noodles to the wok and heat through.

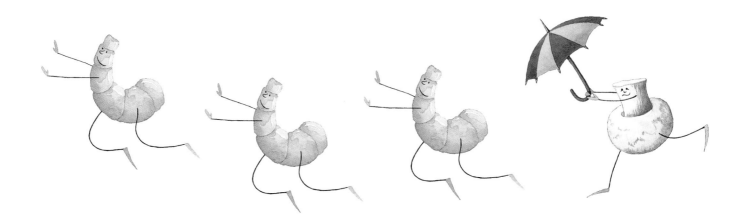

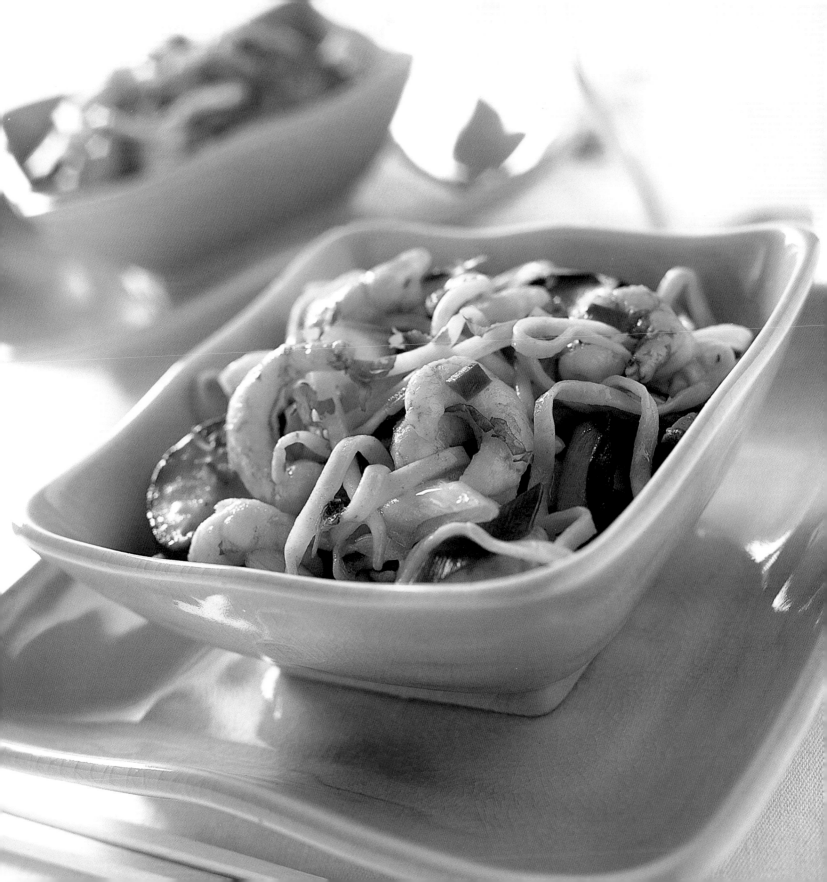

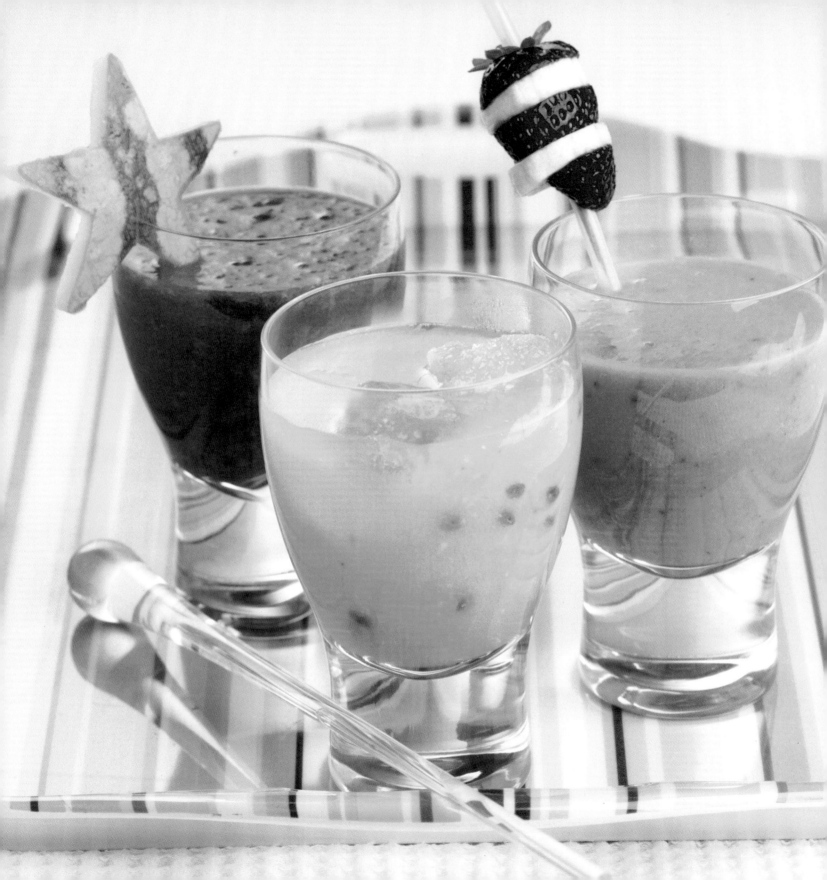

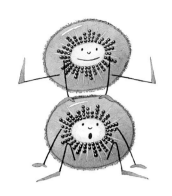

Low-Fat
Recipes

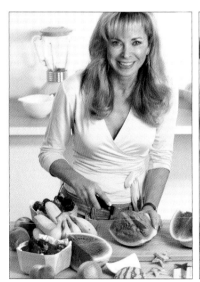
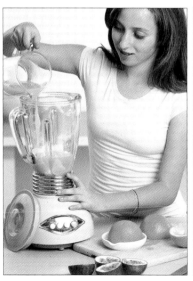
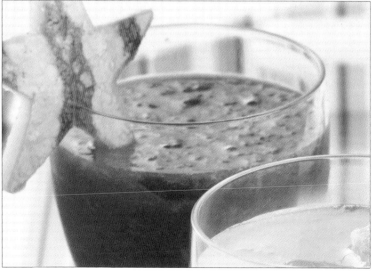

Low-Fat Recipes

Shocking new figures show that one in six ten-year-olds is classed as obese and by the time they reach fifteen, the figure is almost one in five. Obesity in children has doubled in the last twenty years, but it's no surprise when today's children not only eat more junk food but are also becoming less and less active.

Children who are overweight face a greater risk of developing a serious illness such as heart disease, diabetes, or cancer. Children as young as eight are showing signs of heart disease and ten-year-olds are developing the type of diabetes once found only in adults. Around one in eleven deaths is now linked to carrying excess fat and is being blamed on the rise of aggressively marketed fat-laden foods and couch-potato lifestyles. Overweight children suffer both physically and emotionally, and those who remain heavy in adolescence tend to stay that way into adulthood.

FOODS TO AVOID

Fast foods, pre-prepared meals, and sugary, fizzy drinks are high in calories, fats, salt, and sugar, and low in essential nutrients. Sadly, most children eat less than half the recommended five portions of fruit and vegetables a day. However, children now consume thirty times more soft drinks and five times more candy than they did in 1950. Portion sizes are ballooning, too: Most snacks and sweets are sold in super size for just a few pennies more than standard size. It's important to cut out as much processed junk food from your child's diet as you can, since these are the foods that are high in saturated fat, salt, and sugar.

The types of carbohydrates you give your children affect their energy level, their ability to concentrate, and their appetite. Complex carbohydrates such as whole-grain bread, oatmeal, potatoes, and pasta get broken down into sugar in the blood, slowly providing a steady supply of energy. On the other hand, foods such as refined sugary breakfast cereals, white bread and jam, and chocolate are broken down quickly, rapidly increasing the level of sugar in the blood. This gives a quick burst of energy followed by a drop in sugar levels, leaving a child tired, unable to concentrate, and hungry.

Over half the children in this country eat twice as much salt as they should, and it is estimated that by reducing the amount of salt we eat, 14 percent fewer people would suffer strokes and 10 percent fewer people would suffer a heart attack. About three-quarters of the salt children consume comes from processed foods, so to reduce your child's salt intake you must limit the amount of processed foods, snacks, and fast foods such as pizzas, chicken nuggets, spaghetti, and french fries that your child eats.

HOW TO LOSE WEIGHT

With a healthier diet, a child's weight gain should keep apace of his increasing height. Rather than restrict food, you should change the type of food that you give your child and the way you cook it. Give more fruit and vegetables and broil or bake rather than fry foods.

Remember that fitness is vital, too: Make exercise fun by buying a trampoline or jungle gym for the backyard, or get involved yourself with ball games or family bike rides. Encourage your child to walk or cycle to school, if possible, or take the dog for walks in the park.

Avoid using the term *diet,* or children can end up with eating disorders. What you need to do is to stabilize a child's weight while he grows. The message should be that you want your child to be healthier rather than slimmer.

Many parents who work full-time think that cooking fresh food is too time consuming, but it doesn't have to be. Here are some suggestions for healthy alternatives.

ENCOURAGING CHILDREN TO LOSE WEIGHT

✔ It is not good for your child to go to school on an empty stomach. Try to give your child a high-fiber cereal such as oatmeal or shredded wheat with skimmed milk and some fresh fruit. Boiled or poached eggs with whole-wheat toast are good, too.

✔ When children come home from school, they are usually starving. Have some fresh fruit cut up into pieces or raw vegetable sticks and cherry tomatoes with a tasty dip. Leave snacks like these on a low shelf in the refrigerator where children can help themselves.

✔ Charbroiling food on a ridged pan is a tasty way to prepare chicken, fish, and meat and uses minimal oil.

✔ Instead of french fries, offer high-fiber potato skins. If serving french fries, choose low-fat oven fries; the thick-cut variety absorbs less oil.

✔ If vegetables are not popular, try a new approach—stir-fries with soy sauce and noodles; blend vegetables into a tomato sauce for pasta; make a tomato soup with fresh tomatoes, onions, and carrots; or find a salad dressing that your child really likes.

✔ Try to include as much fruit as possible: Add fruit to breakfast cereals or make fruit smoothie combinations such as peach, banana, and strawberry. Desserts such as cakes or ice cream should be a treat rather than the norm. For variety, present fruit in different ways;

for example, serve kiwifruit in an eggcup. You can also make delicious ice pops by pureeing fruit and mixing it with pure fruit juice.

✔ Serve more complex carbohydrates such as baked potatoes, muesli or oatmeal, whole-grain bread, and vegetables. These are absorbed more slowly into the bloodstream than simple carbohydrates such as white rice, sugary refined breakfast cereals, and cakes and cookies, thus providing a more constant supply of energy.

✔ Serve healthy snacks: Popcorn, pretzels, or rice cakes are a good alternative to potato chips. Instead of candy or chocolate bars, give healthy snacks such as pita bread filled with tuna or chicken salad. Pumpkin or sunflower seeds sprinkled with a little soy sauce and honey and broiled for a few minutes make a nutritious, tasty snack.

✔ Cut down on sugary drinks, but be careful about substituting fruit juices; they may be healthier but they also contain high levels of sugar. Encourage your child to drink water.

✔ Cut out between-meal snacks such as potato chips or chocolate cookies and offer healthy foods instead such as fresh fruit or raw vegetables and a dip.

✔ Don't buy foods that you don't want your child to eat. In a house where there is only fruit for dessert, your child is more likely to eat fruit if there isn't chocolate cake in the refrigerator.

Penne with Tuna and Tomato Sauce

The red onion and sun-dried tomatoes give this pasta dish a lovely flavor.

Makes 4 servings

8 ounces penne
2 tablespoons light olive oil
1 medium red onion, sliced
4 ripe plum tomatoes, peeled, quartered, seeded,
and roughly chopped

One 6-ounce can of tuna in oil, drained
3 ounces sun-dried tomatoes, chopped
1 tablespoon balsamic vinegar
Small handful of basil leaves, torn
Salt and freshly ground black pepper

Cook the penne in lightly salted boiling water according to the package instructions. Heat the olive oil in a frying pan and sauté the onion for about 6 minutes, stirring occasionally, until softened. Stir in the fresh tomatoes and cook for 2 to 3 minutes, until heated through and beginning to soften into the onion. Add the tuna, sun-dried tomatoes, balsamic vinegar, basil, and salt and pepper and heat for 1 minute before stirring into the pasta.

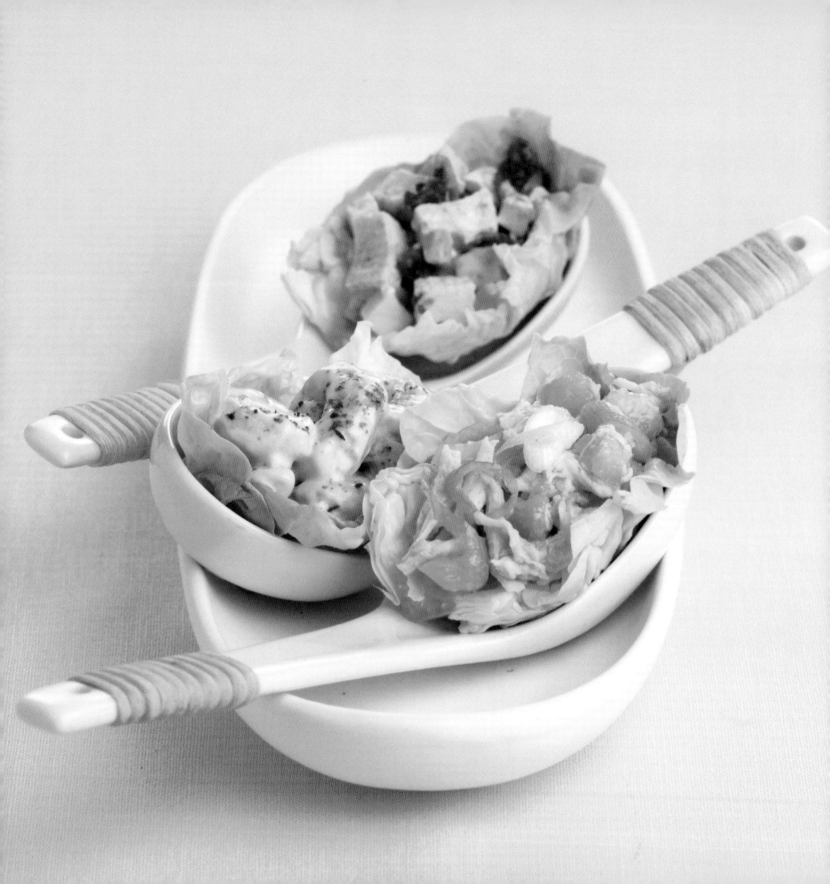

Little Lettuce Cups

Instead of making sandwiches, why not use leaves of Boston lettuce to hold delicious fillings?

Makes 6 little lettuce cups

Chicken and Mango Cups

6 lettuce leaves
³/₄ cup shredded cooked chicken breast
³/₄ cup chopped ripe mango
½ scallion, finely sliced

1 tablespoon lemon juice
1 teaspoon grated lemon zest
2 teaspoons honey
1½ tablespoons light olive oil

Separate the leaves and lay out on a plate. Mix together the shredded chicken, mango, and scallion in a bowl. Mix together the lemon juice, zest, honey, and olive oil and toss with the chicken mixture. Place a spoonful of the mixture on each lettuce leaf and serve immediately.

Makes 4 little lettuce cups

Shrimp and Watercress Cups

4 ounces peeled cooked small shrimp
2 tablespoons light mayonnaise
1 tablespoon ketchup

Handful of watercress, trimmed and chopped
4 lettuce leaves
Paprika

Mix the shrimp together with the mayonnaise and ketchup and stir in the chopped watercress. Spoon some of the mixture onto each lettuce leaf and sprinkle with a little paprika.

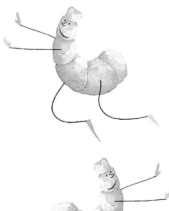

OTHER IDEAS FOR FILLINGS
- Ham, diced pineapple, and cottage cheese
- Diced chicken, corn, light mayonnaise, and scallion
- Diced broiled chicken, salsa, and low-fat sour cream
- Diced chicken, light mayonnaise mixed with a little mild curry powder, and a few raisins
- Shredded chicken, chopped tomato, chopped hard-boiled egg, alfalfa sprouts, and mayonnaise
- Diced turkey, sun-dried tomato, diced avocado, and a little salad dressing or mayonnaise
- Grated carrots, raisins, and light mayonnaise
- Diced cherry tomatoes, mozzarella, and basil with olive oil and balsamic vinegar
- Canned tuna in water mixed with low-fat sour cream, a little ketchup, and sliced scallions
- Canned tuna in water mixed with chopped hard-boiled egg, corn, scallion, some light mayonnaise, and a little white wine vinegar

Stir-fried Chicken with Broccoli

Stir-frying in a wok is a quick and easy method of cooking. Children tend to like Chinese food, so making easy versions in your own kitchen can encourage children to enjoy eating vegetables. It is good to introduce new vegetables such as shiitake mushrooms, which have a lovely flavor.

Makes 4 servings

2 boneless, skinless chicken breasts, cut into strips
Salt
1 tablespoon sake (rice wine)
1½ teaspoons cornstarch
2½ tablespoons vegetable oil
1 clove garlic, crushed
1 medium onion, thinly sliced

1 medium carrot, peeled and cut into matchsticks
1 cup small broccoli florets
3 ounces shiitake mushrooms, finely sliced
¼ cup chicken stock
1 tablespoon oyster sauce
½ teaspoon superfine sugar
Freshly ground black pepper

Season the strips of chicken with a little salt. Mix together the sake and cornstarch, toss with the strips of chicken, and set aside.

Heat 1 tablespoon of the oil in a wok, add half the garlic and the chicken, and stir-fry for 2 minutes. Remove the chicken to a bowl and set aside.

Heat the remaining 1½ tablespoons oil, add the remaining garlic, the onion, and carrot, and stir-fry for 3 minutes. Add the broccoli and mushrooms and stir-fry for 4 minutes.

Mix together the chicken stock, oyster sauce, and sugar. Return the chicken to the wok, add the sauce, and stir-fry for 1 minute. Season to taste.

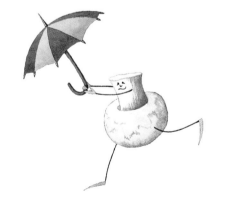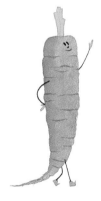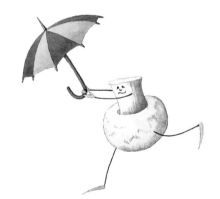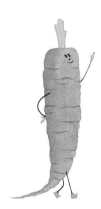

Mini Minute Steaks

This marinade is delicious and will also work well if you marinate cubes of round steak on a skewer
and then cook them in a preheated broiler or on a griddle pan or barbecue.
Red meat is the best and most easily absorbed source of iron, which is often lacking in children's diets.
By preparing meat yourself you can be sure to choose good lean cuts of beef.

Makes 2 servings

1 tablespoon brown sugar
1 tablespoon soy sauce
1½ teaspoons lime or lemon juice
Two 4½-ounce minute steaks (very thin steaks)
1 tablespoon vegetable oil, plus extra
for the griddle pan
1 clove garlic, crushed

1 medium carrot, peeled and cut into matchsticks
2 small zucchini, cut into matchsticks
3 scallions, thinly sliced
¾ cup bean sprouts
¼ cup beef stock
½ teaspoon cornstarch
1 tablespoon oyster sauce

Mix together the sugar, soy sauce, and lime or lemon juice. Add the steaks and leave to marinate for at least 30 minutes.

Remove the steaks and reserve the marinade. Heat the vegetable oil in a wok and stir-fry the garlic for a few seconds. Add the carrot and stir-fry for 2 minutes. Add the zucchini, scallions, and bean sprouts and stir-fry for 2 minutes. Mix a little of the beef stock with the cornstarch to make a paste and then stir in the remaining beef stock and the oyster sauce. Add to the vegetables together with the reserved marinade, bring to a boil, and cook for 1 minute, until thickened slightly.

Brush a griddle pan with a few drops of vegetable oil. Pat the marinated steaks dry with some paper towels and cook the steaks on the griddle for just under 1 minute on each side. Serve with the stir-fried vegetables and sauce.

Honey and Soy Salmon with Sesame

Not all fats are bad. The essential fatty acids in oily fish such as salmon are good for boosting brain power—omega-3 essential fats optimize messaging between nerve cells in the brain. Good intakes are crucial for normal brain functioning and can be of particular benefit to dyslexic and hyperactive children.

Makes 2 servings

2 tablespoons soy sauce
2 tablespoons honey
1 tablespoon rice wine vinegar
2 salmon fillets (approximately 5 ounces each)
1 tablespoon vegetable oil

1 small onion, sliced
3 ounces green beans, trimmed
2 small zucchini, cut into matchsticks
1 heaping teaspoon toasted sesame seeds (dry-fry them over medium heat, stirring until lightly golden)

Mix together the soy sauce, honey, and rice wine vinegar. Place the salmon fillets in a dish and pour over the marinade. Leave to marinate for about 45 minutes. Preheat the broiler. Remove the fish from the marinade and place on a broiler pan. Broil for about 5 minutes, brushing with the marinade halfway through. Meanwhile, heat the oil in a wok and stir-fry the onion for 2 minutes. Add the beans and stir-fry for 4 minutes. Add the zucchini and stir-fry for 3 minutes. Add the remaining marinade from the salmon and continue to stir-fry for about 30 seconds. Sprinkle half the toasted sesame seeds over the stir-fried vegetables. Sprinkle the remaining sesame seeds over the salmon and serve with the vegetables.

Marinated Griddled Chicken

Cooking on a griddle is an excellent way to cook without using very much fat. You can also cook salmon, tuna, steak, or vegetables on the griddle. Always heat the griddle pan before you start cooking: This should take 2 to 3 minutes over medium to high heat. Once the food has seared and a crust has formed, turn down the heat a little to ensure it cooks all the way through. Try this dish with thin slices of zucchini, brushed with oil and griddled for a few minutes on each side.

Makes 2 servings

1½ tablespoons soy sauce
1½ teaspoons light olive oil
1 tablespoon brown sugar
1 tablespoon lemon juice

1 small clove garlic, chopped
2 boneless, skinless chicken breasts
Vegetable oil

Mix together the soy sauce, olive oil, sugar, lemon juice, and garlic in a bowl. Cover the chicken with plastic wrap and bang with a mallet to flatten slightly. Add the chicken to the marinade and leave for 30 minutes to an hour. Remove the chicken from the marinade, strain, and reserve. Heat a griddle pan, brush with a little vegetable oil, and cook the chicken for about 3 minutes on each side or until cooked through. Pour the strained marinade into a small saucepan, bring to a boil, and simmer for 1 minute. Serve the chicken with the sauce.

Tropical Smoothie

Making smoothies for children is a great way to encourage them to consume valuable nutrients. Older children will enjoy blending the fruit themselves and making up their own combinations using fresh or frozen fruits, pure fruit juices, and low-fat yogurt (see photograph, page 104).

Makes 2 glasses

½ large mango, peeled and pitted
4 ounces fresh pineapple (⅛ whole pineapple, peeled and cored), or 1 small banana

1 cup freshly squeezed orange juice
2 tablespoons honey
2 passion fruits (optional)

Cut the mango and pineapple into cubes and blend together with the orange juice and honey. If using, cut the passion fruits in half, scoop out the flesh and seeds, press through a sieve, and add the juice and a few of the seeds to the orange juice mixture. Serve in glasses over ice.

Fruit Salad Smoothie

If you have time, freeze the banana already peeled in a plastic bag with the air pressed out.

Makes 2 glasses

1 cup quartered strawberries
1 banana, sliced (can be frozen first)
1 large ripe peach, peeled, pitted, and cut into pieces

6 ounces low-fat strawberry yogurt drink
½ cup freshly squeezed orange juice

Simply whizz all the ingredients together in a blender.

Watermelon and Strawberry Refresher

This is good to make with blood oranges when they are in season.

Makes 2 glasses

2 cups watermelon cubes
1 cup halved strawberries

Juice of 3 oranges
Sugar

Simply blend together the watermelon, strawberries, and orange juice and sweeten with sugar to taste.

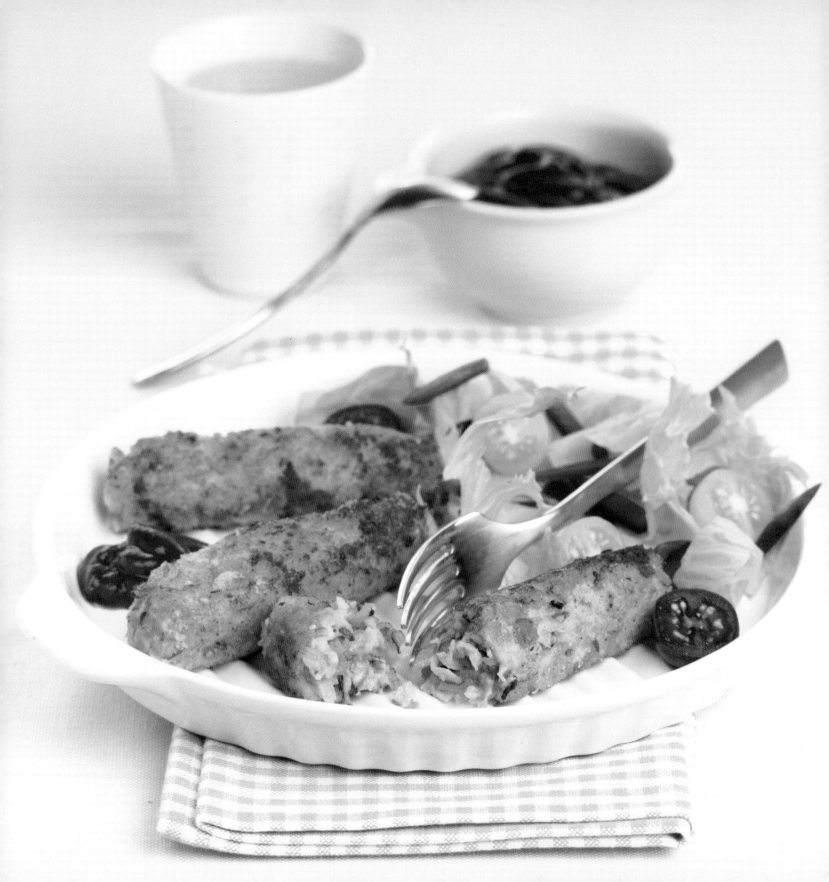

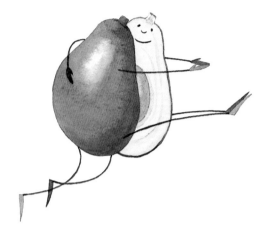

Vegetarian Dishes

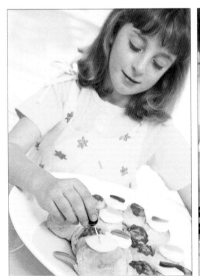
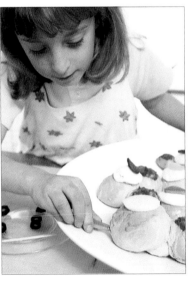
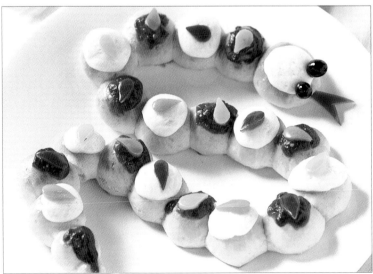

Perfect Chinese Fried Rice

This tends to be very popular with children and can be served as an accompaniment to many of the recipes in this book.

Makes 4 servings

1¼ cups basmati rice
1 small carrot, peeled and finely chopped
¾ cup frozen peas
1 teaspoon vegetable oil
1 egg, lightly beaten
Salt

2 tablespoons butter
½ cup finely chopped onion
2 tablespoons soy sauce
Freshly ground black pepper
1 scallion, finely sliced

Cook the rice in 2½ cups of lightly salted boiling water, together with the chopped carrot, according to the instructions on the package. Four minutes before the end of the cooking time, add the frozen peas. Meanwhile, heat the vegetable oil in a frying pan or wok, beat the egg together with a little salt, and add to the pan. Tilt the pan so that the egg coats the base, and cook until set as a thin omelet. Remove from the pan, roll up to form a sausage shape, and cut into thin strips. Add the butter to the pan and sauté the onion for 2 minutes. Add the cooked rice mixture, the soy sauce, and a little freshly ground black pepper. Stir-fry the rice for about 2 minutes. Stir in the strips of egg and the scallion and heat through.

Baked Summer Squash with a Cheesy Topping

If your child isn't too keen on eating vegetables, try this tasty recipe. It also makes a delicious accompaniment to an adult meal—it works especially well with poultry.

Makes 4 servings

1 medium summer squash
Salt
1 medium onion, chopped
1 tablespoon chopped fresh parsley
2 tablespoons vegetable oil

One 14-ounce can of chopped tomatoes
1 tablespoon torn fresh basil
Freshly ground black pepper
1 cup grated Cheddar cheese

Peel and halve the squash, scoop out the seeds, and cut into 1-inch cubes. Place in a colander, sprinkle with salt, and leave for about 30 minutes. Rinse under the tap and pat dry.

Preheat the oven to 375°F. Sauté the onion and parsley in the oil until softened, add the tomatoes, and cook for about 4 minutes. Add the squash and basil, simmer for 10 to 15 minutes, and season to taste. Transfer to an ovenproof dish, stir in ¾ cup of the cheese, and sprinkle the remaining cheese on top. Bake in the oven for 30 minutes or until browned.

Cannelloni with Mushrooms and Ricotta

A good way to encourage children to eat more vegetables is to stuff the vegetables inside cannelloni.
Try this tasty mushroom filling or mix some cooked spinach with ricotta, Parmesan, and egg.

Makes 4 or 5 servings

2 tablespoons olive oil
1 medium onion, finely chopped
1 clove garlic, crushed
8 ounces button mushrooms, sliced
8 ounces cremini mushrooms, sliced
1 cup ricotta cheese
½ cup grated Cheddar cheese
½ cup grated Parmesan cheese
1 egg, lightly beaten
Salt and freshly ground black pepper

Béchamel Sauce
2 tablespoons butter
2 tablespoons all-purpose flour
1½ cups milk
½ teaspoon ground nutmeg
Salt and freshly ground black pepper

8 sheets lasagne
2 cups good-quality store-bought tomato sauce

Preheat the oven to 350°F. Heat the oil over medium heat and sauté the onion and garlic for 3 to 4 minutes. Add the mushrooms and sauté until the liquid has evaporated. Remove from the heat and stir in the ricotta, Cheddar, 6 tablespoons of the Parmesan cheese, the beaten egg, and seasoning.

To make the béchamel sauce, melt the butter in a pan over low heat. Stir in the flour and cook for 1 minute. Gradually whisk in the milk and nutmeg and season to taste.

Cover the sheets of pasta in boiling water and leave for 5 minutes. Drain, then spoon some of the mushroom filling along the center of each sheet and fold in the two sides.

Spoon 1 cup of the tomato sauce onto the bottom of a suitable ovenproof dish or prepare two smaller dishes and freeze one. Line up the filled tubes next to each other on top of the sauce. Cover with the remaining 1 cup tomato sauce and then spread the béchamel sauce on top. Sprinkle with the remaining 2 tablespoons Parmesan cheese. Bake for 25 to 30 minutes.

ANTIOXIDANTS

Vitamins A, C, and E are known as antioxidants. They are thought to help protect against free radicals, destructive molecules that damage cells and DNA. If left unchecked, these unstable and potentially harmful chemicals can create conditions that may precipitate heart disease and cancer.

Summer Risotto

I like to make my risotto in a large frying pan. You will need to add the liquid to the rice little by little, waiting to add more until all the liquid has been absorbed and stirring frequently. It usually takes about 30 minutes to prepare, depending on your pan and stove. Stir in a little extra stock if you need to reheat the risotto.

Makes 4 to 6 servings

3 cups vegetable or chicken stock
1 tablespoon olive oil
3 tablespoons butter
4 large shallots or 1 medium onion, finely chopped
1 clove garlic, crushed
½ sweet red pepper, chopped

1 cup arborio (risotto) rice
1 small zucchini, diced
2 medium tomatoes, peeled, seeded, and chopped
¼ cup white wine
6 tablespoons grated Parmesan cheese
Salt and freshly ground black pepper

Bring the stock to a boil and allow to simmer. Heat the oil and butter in a large frying pan and sauté the shallots and garlic for 1 minute. Add the red pepper and cook for 5 minutes, stirring occasionally, until softened. Add the rice and stir for 1 minute to make sure that it is well coated. Add 1 or 2 ladlefuls of hot stock and simmer, stirring, until it has been absorbed, then add another ladleful of stock. Continue adding the stock a little at a time and simmer until the rice absorbs the liquid before adding more, stirring frequently. After 10 minutes, add the diced zucchini and the tomatoes. After about 8 minutes add the white wine. When all the stock has been added and the rice is cooked (it will probably take about 20 minutes for the rice to cook through), stir in the Parmesan cheese until melted and season to taste.

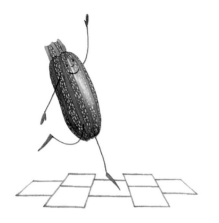
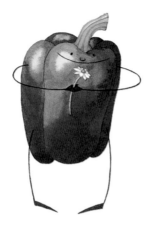
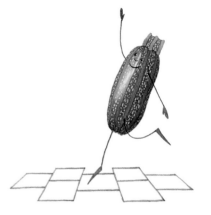

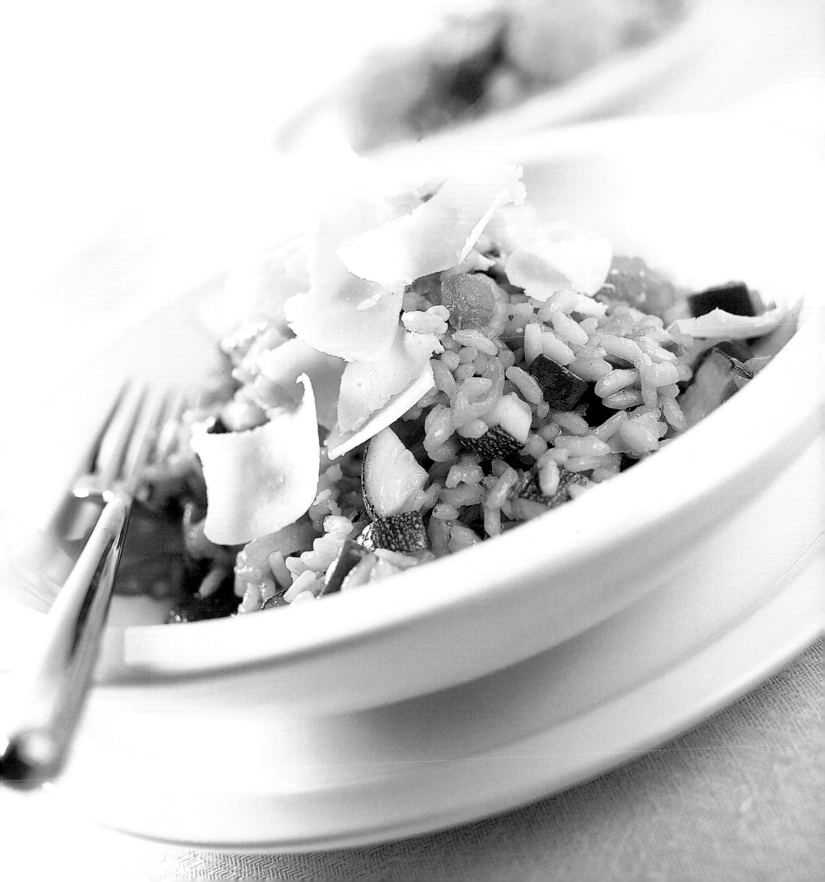

Perfect Baked Potatoes

The best potatoes to choose are floury varieties such as Idaho. You can also make mini baked potatoes by using new potatoes, in which case the cooking time will be shorter. You can also try making baked sweet potatoes and serve these with butter and a little freshly ground black pepper.

Makes 4 servings

4 baking potatoes
Olive oil (optional)

Salt and freshly ground black pepper
1 stick cold butter

Preheat the oven to 400°F. Wash and dry the potatoes and prick the skins a few times with a fork. If you want extra-crisp skins, then rub the skins with a few drops of olive oil and sprinkle with a little salt before baking. Place on the center shelf in the oven for 1 to 1½ hours (the cooking time will depend on the size of the potatoes). To check if the potatoes are cooked, squeeze gently to see if they feel soft. Alternatively, cook in the microwave (see below).

Cut a cross in the top of each potato and squeeze the sides to open them up. Sprinkle with a little salt and freshly ground black pepper and top with butter. Alternatively, cut each of the potatoes in half lengthwise and scoop out the flesh and mash with a little milk, butter, and seasoning.

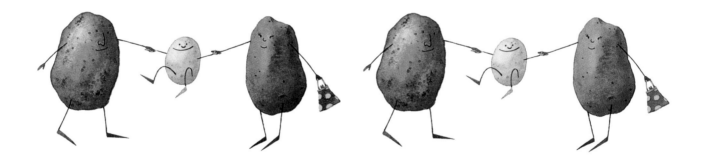

TO MICROWAVE

Prick the potatoes as usual and wrap each one in paper towels. Cook on high for 6 to 7 minutes for 1 potato or about 12 minutes for 2 potatoes and 18 to 20 minutes for 4 potatoes (timing will differ, depending on the size of the potatoes).

OTHER GOOD TOPPINGS

Sour cream and chives
Plain or curried baked beans
Tuna, mayonnaise, and corn
Crisp bacon, scallions, and sour cream
Broccoli and grated cheese
Smoked ham and grated Cheddar cheese

Fluffy Baked Potatoes

Makes 4 servings

4 baked potatoes
4 tablespoons butter
3 tablespoons heavy cream or milk

2 eggs, separated
¾ cup grated Cheddar cheese
Salt and freshly ground black pepper

Preheat the oven to 375°F. Cut each potato in half and scoop out the flesh into a large saucepan, leaving enough around the sides so that they still retain their shape. Add the butter, cream or milk, egg yolks, and ½ cup of the cheese to the potato flesh. Mash together until smooth and season to taste. Whisk the egg whites until stiff and fold into the potato mixture. Carefully spoon this back into the potato skins and sprinkle with the remaining ¼ cup grated cheese. Bake in the oven for 15 minutes, until golden. Serve immediately.

Mini Baked Potatoes

For a change, how about making mini baked potatoes using new potatoes. The potato's best source of fiber and nutrients is in the skin and in the flesh just under the skin. Potatoes are a good source of carbohydrates, which provide energy, and are also a useful and cheap source of vitamin C.

Makes 4 servings

1 pound new potatoes
1 tablespoon olive oil
1 teaspoon dried mixed herbs
2 teaspoons coarse sea salt

Toppings
Sour cream and chives
Crisp bacon, crumbled and mixed with grated cheese and mayonnaise
Tuna salad and corn
Baked beans
Cottage cheese with chives

Preheat the oven to 400°F. Scrub and dry the potatoes. Prick the skins with a fork and mix them with the olive oil and herbs, tossing them in a bowl to coat. Place the potatoes on a baking sheet and sprinkle with the sea salt. Bake for 25 to 30 minutes or until they are crisp and tender. Cut a cross in the top of each potato, squeeze the sides gently to open them up, and fill with a topping of your choice or just simply with some butter.

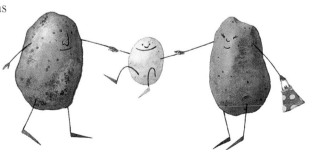

Gratin of Zucchini

This has a light soufflé-type consistency and makes a delicious light lunch with a salad. It can be served as a tasty accompaniment to a meal and looks elegant enough for a dinner party (see photograph).

Makes 6 servings

3 tablespoons vegetable oil
1 pound zucchini, thinly sliced
Salt and freshly ground black pepper
2 tablespoons chopped fresh parsley

4 eggs
½ cup sour cream
1 cup grated Swiss cheese

Preheat the oven to 350°F. Heat the oil in a frying pan and season the zucchini with some salt and freshly ground black pepper. Sauté together with the parsley over low heat for about 20 minutes or until softened. Using a fork, beat the eggs, then beat in the sour cream, Swiss cheese, and a little seasoning. Stir in the zucchini and spoon the mixture into an 8- or 9-inch square ovenproof dish and bake in the oven for 20 to 25 minutes.

Zucchini Fritters

If your children aren't keen on eating vegetables, then try these. They are delicious and were very popular with my tasting panel—even the confirmed vegetable haters.

Makes 4 servings

1 pound zucchini
Salt and freshly ground black pepper
¼ cup cornstarch

½ cup all-purpose flour
Vegetable oil for deep frying

Wash and dry the zucchini and trim the ends. Cut them into sticks about 2¼ inches long and ¾ inches wide and season with salt and pepper. Beat together the cornstarch and flour with 1 cup of water and some salt and pepper to form a thin batter.

Heat the oil in a deep-fat fryer with a basket filled with oil to a depth of about 2 inches. Alternatively, you can use a heavy pan and a metal slotted spoon or strainer. Heat the oil until it reaches a temperature of 375°F (you can tell when it is hot enough for frying if a piece of vegetable sizzles as it touches the oil). Dip the zucchini sticks into the batter and fry them until crispy and golden. Lift out the basket or remove the zucchini fritters with a slotted spoon or strainer. Drain on paper towels and serve immediately.

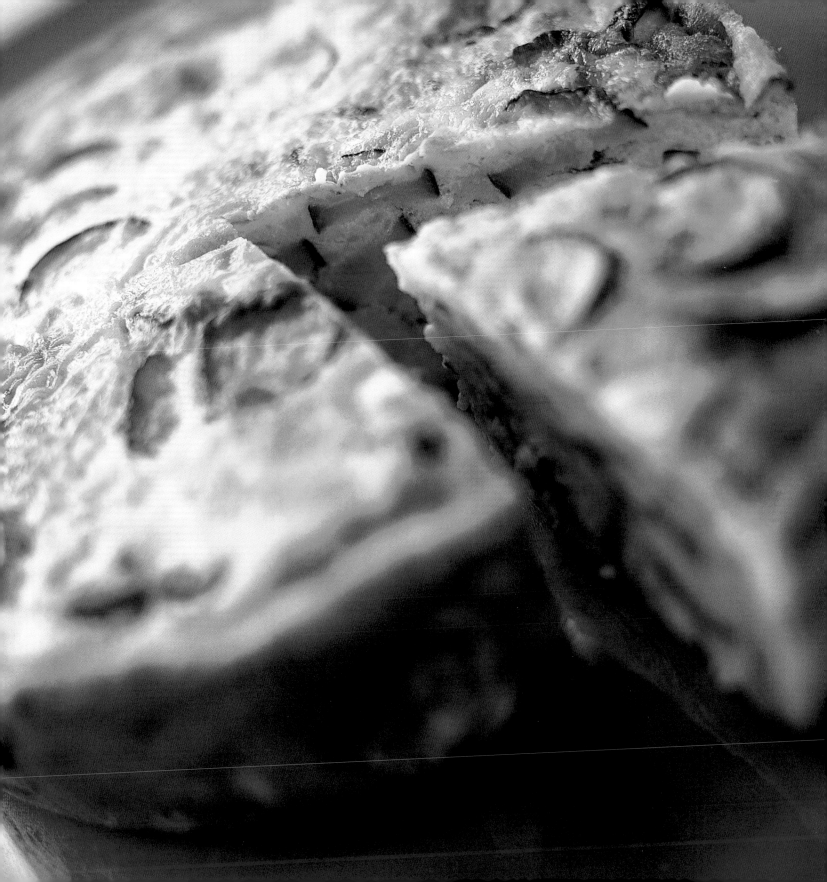

Super Vegetarian Spring Rolls

Spring rolls are actually quite easy to make and children love them. These are filled with vegetables and rice noodles and are bound to be a great hit! Spring rolls can be frozen and reheated in a hot oven.

Makes 24 spring rolls

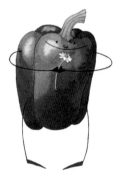

2 tablespoons vegetable oil, plus extra for deep frying
1 medium onion, sliced
1 clove garlic, crushed
1 medium carrot, peeled and cut into thin strips
½ sweet red pepper, cut into thin strips
1½ cups shredded white cabbage
1 cup bean sprouts
8 button mushrooms, thinly sliced
2 scallions, finely sliced
3 ounces fine rice noodles
1 tablespoon cornstarch
1 tablespoon oyster sauce

1½ teaspoons soy sauce
1 teaspoon sugar
1 vegetable stock cube
24 spring roll wrappers
1 egg, lightly beaten

Dipping Sauce
¼ cup rice wine vinegar
1 tablespoon brown sugar
¼ cup sake (rice wine)
1 tablespoon soy sauce
½ red chile, seeded and finely sliced
1 tablespoon finely sliced scallion (optional)

Heat the oil in a wok or frying pan and stir-fry the onion and garlic until lightly golden. Add the carrot and sweet red pepper and stir-fry for 3 minutes. Add the cabbage, bean sprouts, mushrooms, and scallions and stir-fry for 3 to 4 minutes. Cook the rice noodles according to the instructions on the package and then rinse in a colander under cold water. Cut the noodles into short lengths of about 1 inch. Stir the cornstarch into 1 tablespoon of water and combine with the oyster sauce, soy sauce, and sugar. Add the noodles to the vegetables in the wok, pour in the sauce, and crumble over the stock cube. Stir-fry, mixing everything together, for 2 minutes.

Fold over one corner of each spring roll wrapper. Place 2 to 3 tablespoons of the filling about one-third of the way down. Roll over once, fold in both ends, and roll over to form a spring roll. Brush the remaining corner with some beaten egg and press down to seal. To cook the spring rolls, heat vegetable oil in a wok or deep fryer until hot, then reduce the heat. Deep-fry the spring rolls in batches for 2 to 3 minutes or until lightly golden and crispy, then remove and drain on paper towels.

To make the dipping sauce, place the vinegar and sugar in a pan and dissolve the sugar over gentle heat. Bring to a boil and simmer for 3 minutes, until slightly reduced. Add the sake and bring to a boil, then remove from the heat and stir in the soy sauce. Allow to cool down a little and then stir in the chile and scallion, if using.

Cheesy Vegetable Sausages

If you are finding it difficult to get your child to enjoy eating vegetables, try these delicious vegetarian sausages, which are quick and easy to prepare. If you have time, you can form the mixture into sausage shapes and then set them aside in the refrigerator to firm up before frying (see photograph, page 114).

Makes 8 sausages

3 slices of white bread
½ cup grated carrot
1 cup grated zucchini
2 tablespoons butter
1 medium onion, finely chopped

1 cup grated Cheddar cheese
1 egg, separated
Salt and freshly ground black pepper
Vegetable oil

Make the bread crumbs by tearing the bread into pieces and blitzing it in a food processor. Squeeze the excess liquid out of the carrot and zucchini.

Heat the butter in a frying pan and fry the onion until soft. Add the grated carrot and cook for 2 minutes. Add the zucchini and cook for 3 minutes, until softened. Transfer the vegetables to a bowl and mix with the grated cheese, half the bread crumbs, the egg yolk, and a little seasoning.

Shape into 8 sausages about 4 inches long, using floured hands. Dip into the lightly beaten egg white and then roll in the remaining bread crumbs. Heat some oil in a wok or frying pan and panfry the sausages until lightly golden.

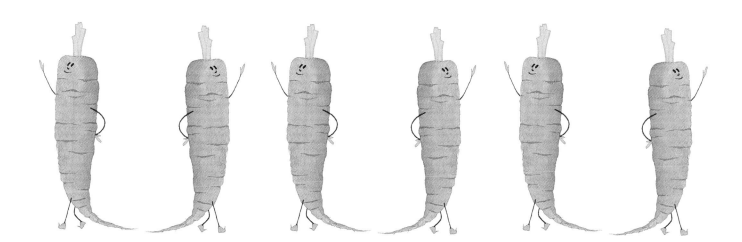

Caramelized Onion and Swiss Tart

This is my favorite recipe for quiche, and the slow cooking of the onions gives them a delicious flavor. The pastry takes only a few minutes to make in a food processor, but you can use store-bought short crust pastry instead.

Makes 8 servings

Pastry
1½ cups all-purpose flour
Pinch of salt
½ teaspoon ground mustard
1 stick butter, diced
3 tablespoons cold water

Filling
1 tablespoon vegetable oil
1 tablespoon butter
1 pound onions, thinly sliced
Salt and freshly ground black pepper
4 eggs
1 cup milk
1 cup light cream
1 cup grated Swiss cheese

¼ cup grated Parmesan cheese

Place the flour, salt, mustard, and butter in a food processor and process until the mixture resembles soft bread crumbs. Gradually add enough water to form a good consistency. Press into a ball with your hands and chill in the refrigerator for at least 30 minutes.

Preheat the oven to 425°F. To make the filling, heat the vegetable oil and butter in a large frying pan and sauté the onions over fairly high heat for about 5 minutes. Lower the heat and cook for another 20 minutes, covered, and stir occasionally until the onions are caramelized. Season with a little salt. Lightly beat the eggs in a large bowl and stir in the milk, cream, and grated Swiss cheese. Season with a little pepper and stir in the caramelized onions.

Grease a 9-inch loose-bottomed tart pan. On a lightly floured work surface, roll out the dough and line the base and sides of the pan. Prick the base of the pastry, cover with baking paper, fill with dried beans, and bake in the oven for 10 minutes. Remove the baking paper and the beans, reduce the temperature to 375°F, and bake for another 5 minutes. Spoon the onion mixture into the crust and sprinkle with the Parmesan cheese. Bake in the oven for 20 to 25 minutes.

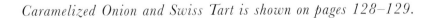

Caramelized Onion and Swiss Tart is shown on pages 128–129.

Vegetable Burgers

These vegetable burgers are delicious eaten either hot or cold.

Makes 8 vegetable burgers

2 medium carrots, peeled and grated
1 medium zucchini, grated
1 medium onion, chopped
¾ cup chopped cremini or button mushrooms
¾ cup roughly chopped cashew nuts
1 tablespoon chopped fresh oregano or
½ teaspoon dried oregano
1 tablespoon chopped fresh parsley

Pinch of cayenne pepper (optional)
2 cups fresh whole-grain bread crumbs
1 tablespoon tomato paste
1½ teaspoons soy sauce
½ lightly beaten small egg
Salt and freshly ground black pepper
Vegetable oil

Using your hands, squeeze out some of the excess moisture from the grated carrots and zucchini. In a large bowl, mix together the vegetables, cashew nuts, herbs, cayenne pepper, if using, and 1 cup of the bread crumbs. Beat together the tomato paste, soy sauce, and egg; stir this into the vegetable mixture and season. Using your hands, form the mixture into 8 burgers and coat with the remaining 1 cup bread crumbs. At this stage you can set the burgers aside in the refrigerator to firm up, but it is not essential. Sauté the burgers in vegetable oil, turning occasionally, until golden.

Mashed Potato with Carrot

There are lots of different ways to turn ordinary mashed potatoes into something special. This is one of my favorites. For a really smooth texture you can add a little more butter and milk. Mashed potato and sweet potato with milk, butter, and a little grated Parmesan cheese is also delicious.

Makes 3 servings

1 pound potatoes, peeled and chopped
1 large carrot, peeled and thinly sliced
1 tablespoon butter

1 tablespoon milk
Salt and freshly ground black pepper

Put the potatoes and carrot into a pot of lightly salted water. Bring to a boil and then cook for about 20 minutes or until the vegetables are tender. Drain and then mash together with the butter, milk, and seasoning until quite smooth. You can make lovely domes of mashed potato using an ice cream scoop.

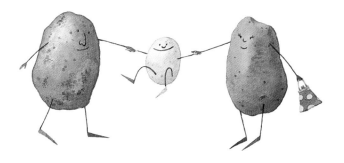

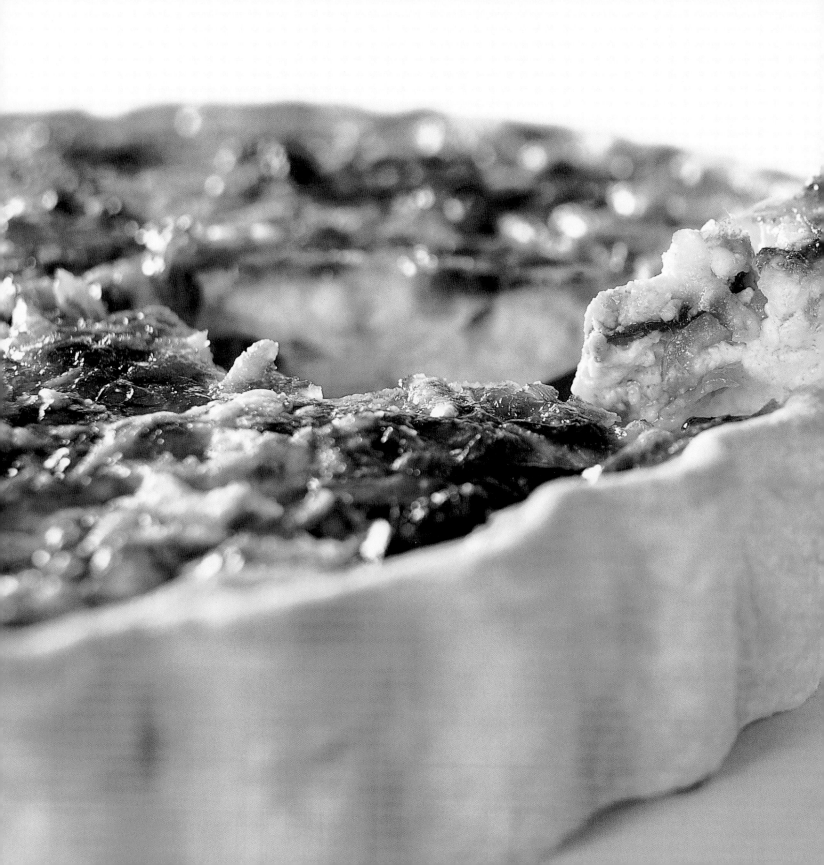

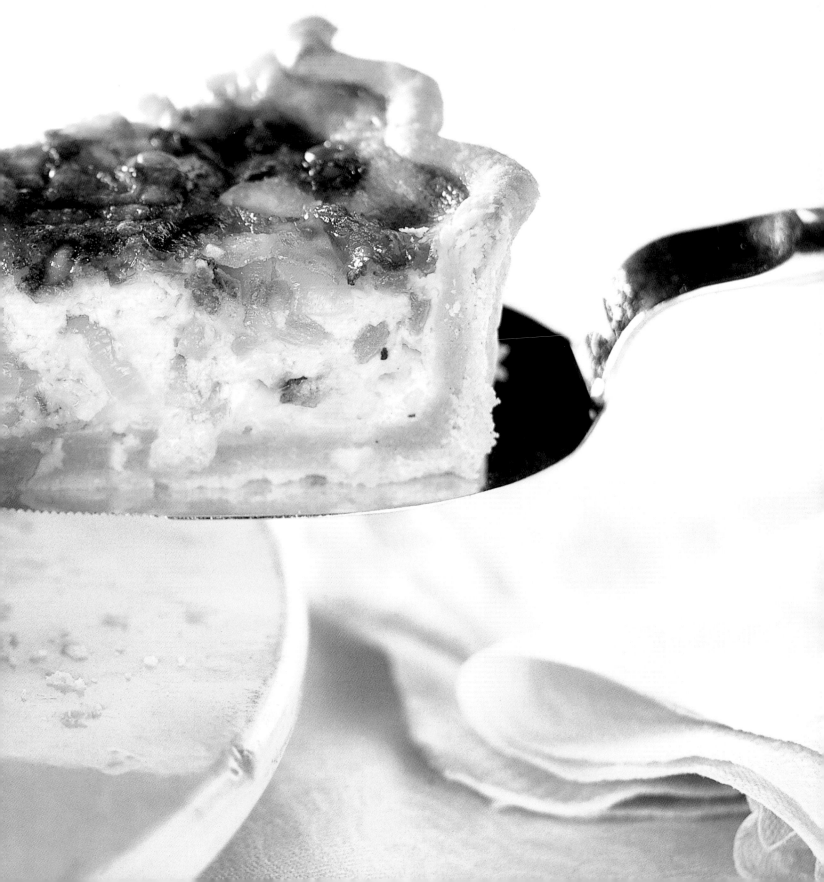

Ratatouille Omelet

This concoction of sautéed Mediterranean vegetables mixed with eggs and topped with grated cheese in the style of a Spanish omelet is quite delicious and a meal in itself (see photograph).

Makes 6 servings

1 small onion, sliced
3 tablespoons olive oil
1 eggplant, sliced
1 large zucchini, sliced
1 sweet red pepper, cored, seeded,
and cut into strips
2 tomatoes, peeled, seeded, and chopped

Salt and freshly ground black pepper
6 eggs
2 tablespoons cold water
2 tablespoons butter
6 tablespoons heavy cream
¾ cup grated Swiss cheese

Gently sauté the onion in the olive oil in a heavy-bottomed frying pan until soft. Chop the eggplant and add with the zucchini and red pepper, cover the pan, and cook for about 20 minutes or until the vegetables are soft but not mushy. Add the tomatoes and cook for another 5 minutes. Season to taste. In a large bowl, lightly whisk the eggs with the cold water, then mix in the cooked vegetables. Heat the butter in a deep 10-inch omelet or frying pan. When the butter is frothy, pour the egg mixture into the pan and cook until set. Remove from the heat, pour over the cream, and cover with the grated cheese. Cook under a preheated broiler for a few minutes, until golden. Leave the handle of the frying pan sticking out of the broiler and cover with foil if necessary.

Delicious Vegetable Rissoles

I make fresh bread crumbs for this recipe by putting two slices of whole-grain bread in a food processor.

Makes 12 rissoles

¾ cup finely chopped leek
Vegetable oil
2 medium carrots, peeled and grated
1 cup grated butternut squash
1½ cups finely chopped button mushrooms

1 tablespoon chopped fresh parsley
1 cup fresh whole-grain bread crumbs
2 teaspoons soy sauce
1 egg, lightly beaten
Salt and freshly ground black pepper

Sauté the leek in a little oil for 2 minutes and squeeze some of the juices from the grated carrots and squash. Mix together with the remaining vegetables, parsley, bread crumbs, soy sauce, beaten egg, and seasoning and chop for a few seconds in a food processor. Using your hands, form into about 12 rissoles. Heat some oil in a large frying pan and sauté the rissoles over medium heat for 8 to 10 minutes, turning occasionally, until golden and cooked through.

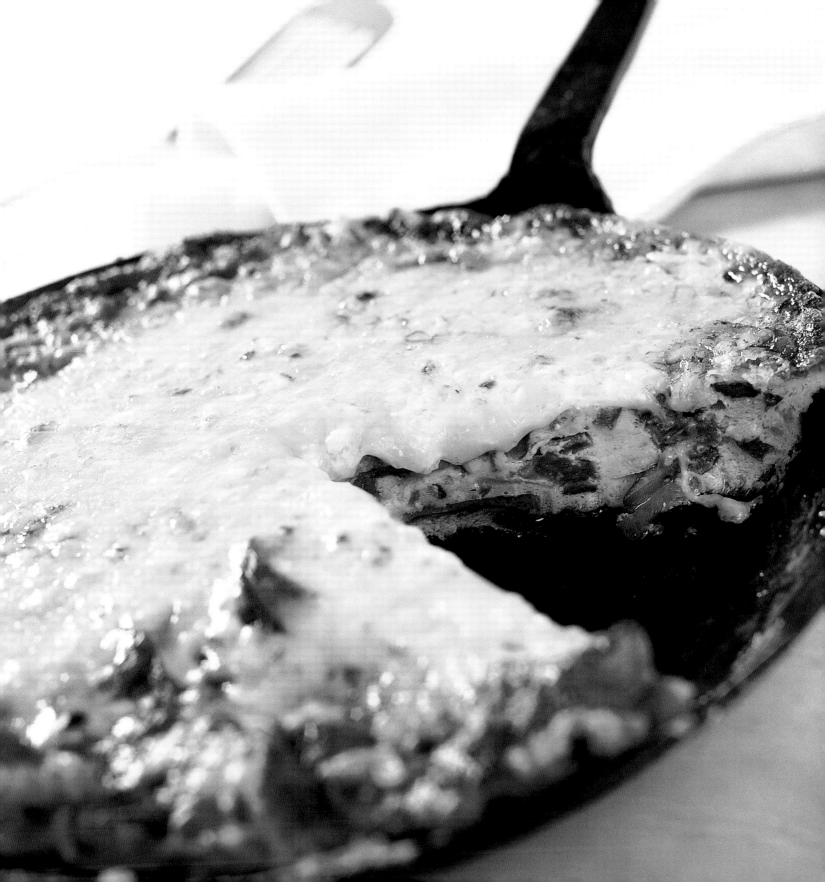

Spotted Snake Pizza

This pizza is great fun to make together with your child. It almost looks too good to eat!

Makes 4 servings

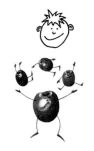

1 tablespoon active dry yeast
Pinch of sugar
2 tablespoons olive oil
3 cups all-purpose flour
1 teaspoon salt
3 ounces Cheddar cheese, cut into 12 cubes
1 egg, lightly beaten

Topping
¾ cup store-bought tomato sauce with herbs
8 ounces mozzarella cheese, cut into slices
Red, orange, and yellow sweet peppers,
cored and seeded
2 black olives, pitted
Small piece of green pepper

Place the yeast in a mixing bowl, add 1 cup of lukewarm water, stir in the sugar, and mix with a fork. Allow to stand until the yeast has dissolved and starts to foam, about 10 minutes. Stir in the olive oil, then mix the flour and salt together and fold half of this mixture into the bowl using a wooden spoon. Gradually mix in three-quarters of the remaining flour, stirring with the spoon until the dough forms a sticky mass and begins to come away from the sides of the bowl.

Sprinkle some of the remaining flour onto a smooth work surface. Remove the dough from the bowl and gradually knead in the remaining flour, a little at a time, until the dough is smooth and elastic and no longer sticks to your hands. This will probably take between 8 and 10 minutes. Form into a ball and place in an oiled bowl, cover with a damp kitchen towel, and leave in a warm place to rise for about 50 minutes, or until doubled in size. To test whether the dough has risen enough, stick two fingers in the dough and if the indentations remain, the dough is ready. Punch the dough down with your fist and place on a floured work surface. Knead again for a few minutes, until the dough is nice and elastic.

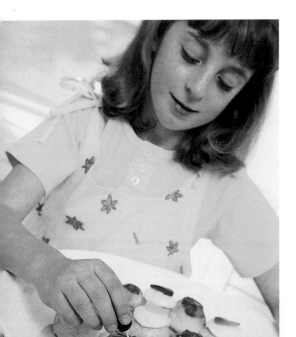

Preheat the oven to 400°F. Divide the dough into about 12 balls with one larger ball for the head of the snake and a small tail made from the dough for the end of the snake. Stuff each of the balls with a small cube of Cheddar cheese, making sure it is completely covered with dough. Place the balls and tail on a large greased baking tray in the shape of a snake so that they are just touching each other. Brush the tops of the balls with the beaten egg and bake in the oven for 10 minutes or until lightly golden and joined together.

Top each ball alternately with tomato sauce and a slice of mozzarella cheese, and decorate with sweet pepper shapes, which can be cut out using mini cookie cutters. Bake for another 5 minutes. Add the olives for eyes and a forked tongue cut from a strip of green pepper to complete the snake.

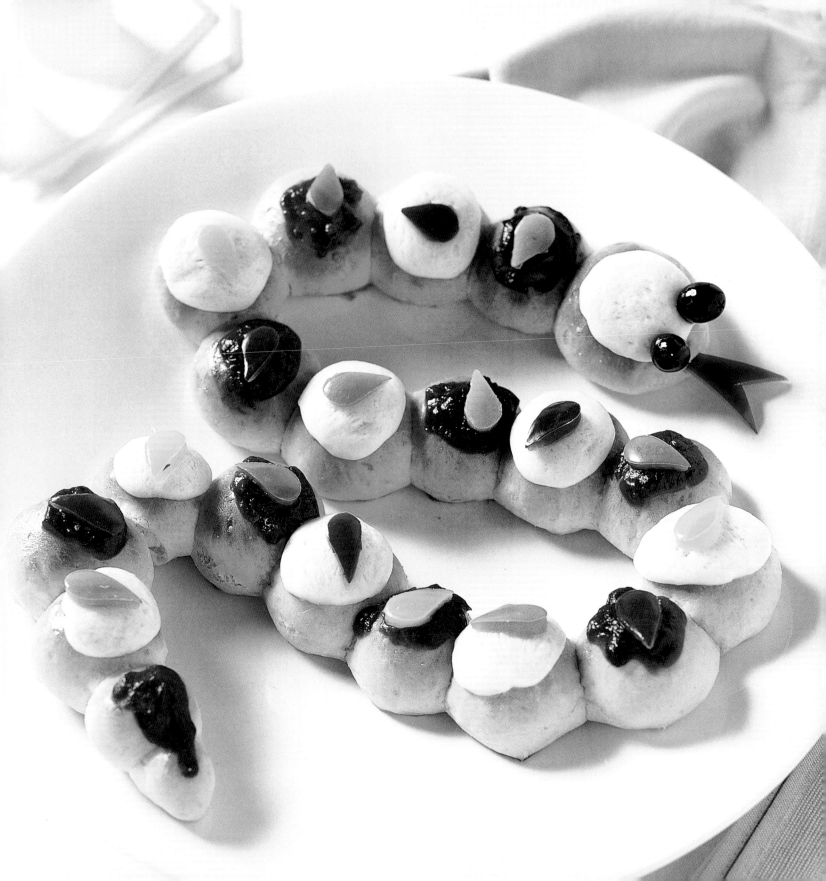

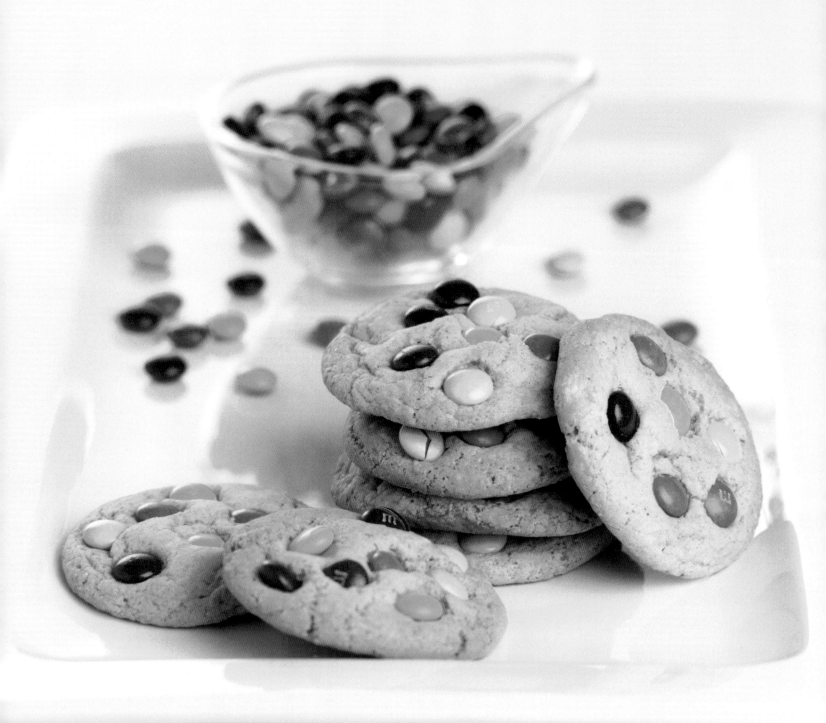

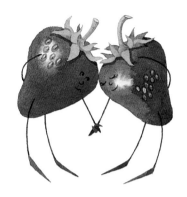

Cakes and Cookies

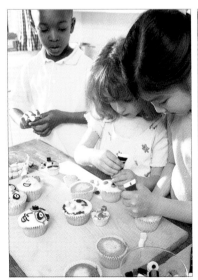

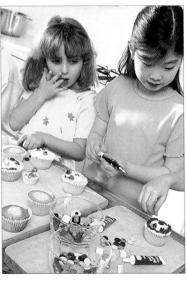

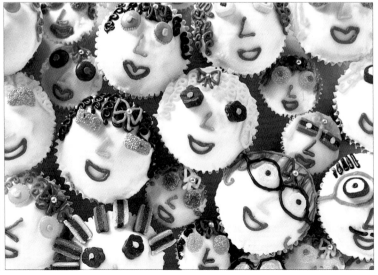

Josie's Delicious Carrot Cake

Carrot cake is one of my favorite cakes, and Josie is a friend of mine who is always keen to try out my new recipes on her husband and two boys. This is her favorite recipe for carrot cake. I've added the chopped pecans, raisins, and marzipan carrots, but you can leave these out if you prefer.

Makes 6 to 8 servings

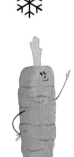

¾ cup vegetable oil
1¼ cups light brown sugar
3 eggs, lightly beaten
1 cup all-purpose flour, sifted
1¼ teaspoons baking powder
1¼ teaspoons baking soda
1 teaspoon salt
1 teaspoon ground cinnamon
¼ teaspoon ground nutmeg
1½ cups grated carrot
½ cup finely chopped pecans
¾ cup raisins

Icing

3 tablespoons unsalted butter, softened
¾ cup confectioners' sugar, sifted
1 teaspoon pure vanilla extract
4 ounces cream cheese

Marzipan Carrots

8 ounces marzipan
Orange and green food coloring

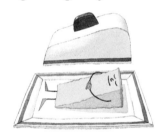

Preheat the oven to 350°F. Grease and line an 8-inch cake pan. Mix the oil and sugar together and add the beaten eggs. Add the flour, baking powder, baking soda, salt, cinnamon, and nutmeg, then stir in the grated carrot, pecans, and raisins. Put the mixture in the prepared pan and bake in the oven for 50 minutes.

To make the icing, beat together the butter, sugar, and vanilla; this is best done with a wooden spoon. Stir in the cream cheese until blended, but don't overbeat or the icing will become watery. When the cake is cool, spread the cream cheese frosting evenly over the top of the cake using a palette knife dipped in warm water. Then use a fork to make decorative swirls in the frosting.

To make the marzipan carrots, divide the marzipan into one large and one small ball. Knead some orange food coloring into the larger ball and knead some green food coloring into the smaller ball. Then mold the marzipan into carrots to decorate the cake.

Poppy Seed and Almond Cake

Dark poppy seeds add lovely texture and flavor to this moist almond sponge cake.

Makes 6 to 8 servings

1 stick plus 2 tablespoons unsalted butter
⅔ cup sugar
2 large eggs
1 cup self-rising flour
½ cup ground almonds

1 teaspoon grated lemon zest
¾ teaspoon almond extract
2 tablespoons very hot water
1 tablespoon poppy seeds

Preheat the oven to 350°F. Grease and line the base of a 7-inch loose-bottomed round tart pan. Beat the butter and sugar together until light and fluffy. Beat in the eggs, one at a time, adding a tablespoon of the flour with the second egg to stop the mixture from curdling. Sift in the flour and ground almonds, add the lemon zest and almond extract, and fold into the mixture. Finally, stir in the hot water and 1½ teaspoons of the poppy seeds. Spoon the mixture into the prepared pan, level the top, and sprinkle with the remaining 1½ teaspoons poppy seeds. Bake in the oven for about 50 minutes or until a skewer inserted in the center of the cake comes out clean. Remove from the pan and allow to cool on a wire rack.

Best-Ever Oatmeal Raisin Cookies

These delicious cookies are made with oats, raisins, and whole-grain flour to give long-lasting energy. Make sure Mommy and Daddy don't gobble them up before the children get some!

Makes about 15 cookies

6 tablespoons unsalted butter or margarine
2 tablespoons brown sugar
2 tablespoons granulated sugar
½ lightly beaten egg
1 teaspoon pure vanilla extract
¼ cup whole-grain flour

½ teaspoon ground cinnamon
or pumpkin pie spice
¼ teaspoon salt
¼ teaspoon baking soda
1½ cups quick-cooking rolled oats
½ cup raisins

Preheat the oven to 350°F. Cream the butter or margarine with the sugars. Beat in the egg and add the vanilla. Sift together the flour, cinnamon, salt, and baking soda. Mix this into the butter mixture. Finally, stir in the oats and raisins. Line 3 baking sheets with nonstick baking paper. Make walnut-size balls of dough and flatten these down onto the baking sheet—you may want to enlist the help of your child for this stage. Bake for about 15 minutes, until the edges are done but the centers are still soft.

Funny Face Cupcakes

These are always very popular at children's birthday parties, decorated with faces made from a mixture of small candies and writing icing. My children adore making their own funny faces. You can also make miniature cupcakes for young children using the small paper cups used for candy and baking the cakes in a mini-muffin tin.

Makes 10 large cupcakes or 24 to 30 mini cupcakes

1 cup self-rising flour
4 tablespoons soft margarine
½ cup superfine sugar
2 eggs
1 teaspoon pure vanilla extract
½ teaspoon grated lemon zest (optional)
½ cup raisins or sultanas (optional)

Icing and Decoration
¾ cup confectioners' sugar
Small tubes of colored writing icing
(available in most supermarkets)
Licorice, gumdrops, and other candies

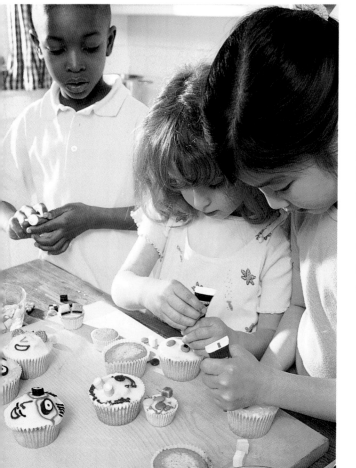

Preheat the oven to 350°F. Put 10 paper liners in a muffin tin or 24 to 30 smaller ones in a mini-muffin tin. Sift the flour into a mixing bowl. Add the margarine, superfine sugar, and eggs and beat everything together until the mixture is soft and creamy. Beat in the vanilla and lemon zest, if using. If you don't want to decorate the cupcakes, you can make plump raisin or sultana cupcakes by folding the raisins or sultanas into the batter at this stage.

Spoon the batter into the liners until about two-thirds full. Bake the larger cupcakes in the oven for about 20 minutes, and the smaller cupcakes for about 12 minutes, or until a toothpick inserted into the center comes out clean. Turn them onto a wire rack to cool.

To make the icing, sift the confectioners' sugar into a bowl and gradually stir in a little water to make a thick smooth paste. Once the cupcakes are cool, ice and decorate them.

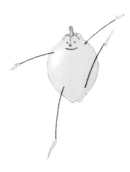

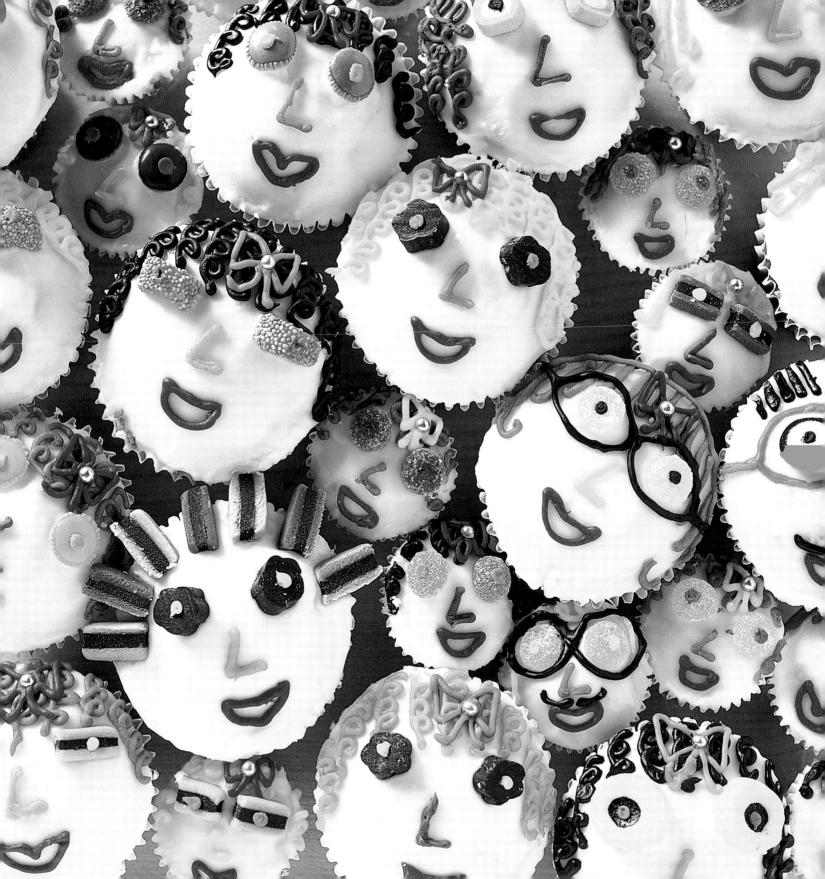

Raspberry Ripple Cheesecake

This is the most fabulous cheesecake. It is easy to make and requires no baking. It is sure to be a great hit!

Makes 8 servings

8 ounces graham crackers
1 stick unsalted butter
2 cups (1 pint) fresh raspberries
½ cup confectioners' sugar

1 pound cream cheese
1½ cups superfine sugar
1 tablespoon pure vanilla extract
1½ cups heavy cream

Break the graham crackers into pieces, place in a plastic bag, and crush with a rolling pin. Melt the butter in a pan and stir in the crushed cookies. Spread the mixture over the base of an 8-inch cake pan and place in the refrigerator.

Put the raspberries into a pan with the confectioners' sugar. Bring to a boil, then lower the heat and simmer for about 8 minutes. Press the raspberries through a sieve to get rid of the seeds. Set aside to cool.

Beat the cream cheese, superfine sugar, and vanilla in a mixer for a couple of minutes. Beat the cream until stiff, but take care not to overbeat. Fold into the cream cheese mixture.

Remove the cake pan from the refrigerator and spread one-third of the cheesecake mixture over the graham cracker base. Swirl a few tablespoons of the raspberry puree into the cheesecake mixture. Spoon half the remaining cheesecake mixture on top and again swirl in a few tablespoons of the raspberry puree. Spread the remaining cheesecake mixture on top and level with a palette knife. Decorate the top of the cake by trailing lines of raspberry puree dropped from a teaspoon horizontally across the cake. Using a skewer, draw vertical lines through the puree to create a pattern.

Refrigerate for at least 2 hours or overnight.

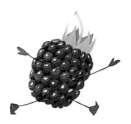
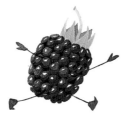
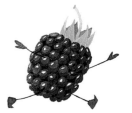

Scrumptious Marble Cake Squares

This not only looks fabulous but tastes great, too! It never lasts long in my house. Children will enjoy helping you make this and swirling the two colored batters together.

Makes 6 to 8 squares

3 ounces milk chocolate or semisweet chocolate, broken into pieces
12 tablespoons unsalted butter
2 ounces white chocolate, broken into pieces

4 eggs
1¼ cups light brown sugar
1¼ cups all-purpose flour, sifted
½ cup plus 2 tablespoons sour cream

Preheat the oven to 350°F. Put the milk or semisweet chocolate and 6 tablespoons of the butter in a heatproof bowl over a pan of simmering water and stir until melted. Set aside to cool. Melt the remaining 6 tablespoons butter together with the white chocolate in a heatproof bowl over a pan of simmering water. Set aside to cool. Beat the eggs and sugar together in an electric mixer for 2 to 3 minutes, until light and fluffy. Transfer half the mixture to another bowl. Stir the milk chocolate mixture into one of the bowls and the white chocolate mixture into the other. Fold half the flour and half the sour cream into each bowl. Place alternate spoonfuls of the mixture in a greased and lined 11 x 7-inch shallow baking pan. Swirl the mixture using a skewer or blunt knife to create a marbled effect and bake in the oven for 30 to 35 minutes. Allow to cool in the pan and then transfer to a wire rack.

SWEET FOODS AND TOOTH DECAY

It is the frequency with which sweet foods are eaten that does the most damage to your child's teeth. It is much better to eat sugary foods or drink fruit juices with a meal or at the end of a meal rather than snack on sweet foods between meals. Once sugar is on the tooth surface, the bacteria in the mouth can produce acids from the sugar and cause dental decay, and the more often sweet foods are eaten, the more chance there is of dental decay. Soft sticky sweets such as toffee, chewy candy, or raisins are particularly damaging.

The saliva in the mouth helps to wash away the sugars, and sugar-free chewing gum is good, as it promotes the production of saliva. If possible, it is best to brush teeth before eating breakfast as well as after breakfast, as it will help remove the bacteria and plaque from the teeth.

Foods high in calcium can help reverse early dental caries. Finishing a meal with cheese or giving cheese as a snack between meals helps to protect your child's teeth from decay. Cheese contains fat and salt to stimulate acid-neutralizing saliva, plus a combination of calcium and a milk protein that speeds up natural repairs to the surface of the teeth. Cheese is also effective against acid from soft drinks and fruit juices such as orange juice (even pure fruit juices contain natural sugars that can damage teeth). Try to limit sweet foods to mealtimes and encourage young children to enjoy eating healthy snacks such as the following:

- Apples • Cheese
- Raw vegetables with a dip or salads
- Rice cakes • Yogurt

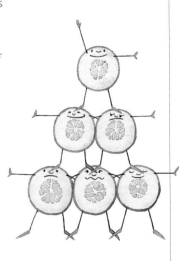

Annabel's Apricot Cookies

This fabulous and rather unusual combination of dried apricots and white chocolate makes irresistible cookies.

Makes 26 cookies

1 stick unsalted butter
4 ounces cream cheese
1 cup superfine sugar
¾ cup all-purpose flour

½ cup chopped dried apricots
½ cup white chocolate chips
or chopped white chocolate

Preheat the oven to 350°F. In a large mixing bowl, cream together the butter and cream cheese. Add the sugar and beat until fluffy. Gradually add the flour, then fold in the apricots and chocolate. The dough will be quite soft—don't worry! Drop the mixture by heaping teaspoons onto baking sheets lined with nonstick baking paper and bake in the oven for 15 minutes or until lightly golden. Allow to cool and harden for a few minutes before removing them from the baking sheets.

Teddy Bear Cupcakes

Try making these for a teddy bear's picnic with sandwiches and cookies cut into teddy bear shapes.

Makes 8 cupcakes

1 stick unsalted butter
⅔ cup superfine sugar
2 eggs, separated
1 teaspoon pure vanilla extract
⅓ cup milk
1¼ cups all-purpose flour
1 teaspoon baking powder
½ teaspoon salt

Decoration
M&M's
Tube of black writing icing
Gumdrops
Chocolate buttons

Preheat the oven to 350°F. Line 8 muffin tin cups with paper liners. Cream the butter and sugar in a food processor until fluffy. Beat in the egg yolks, vanilla, and milk. Transfer the mixture to a large bowl. Sift the flour, baking powder, and salt together, then fold into the butter mixture. Whisk the egg whites in a bowl until stiff, then fold them gently into the batter a little at a time. Fill the liners about two-thirds full. Bake for about 20 minutes or until the tops are golden and spring back when gently pressed or when a toothpick inserted in the center comes out clean. Cool on a wire rack. (Cupcakes may be frozen when cool and decorated at a later time.) To decorate, use the M&M's for eyes and attach with a blob of icing; add a gumdrop for the nose. Fill in the pupils with icing and stick on chocolate buttons for ears.

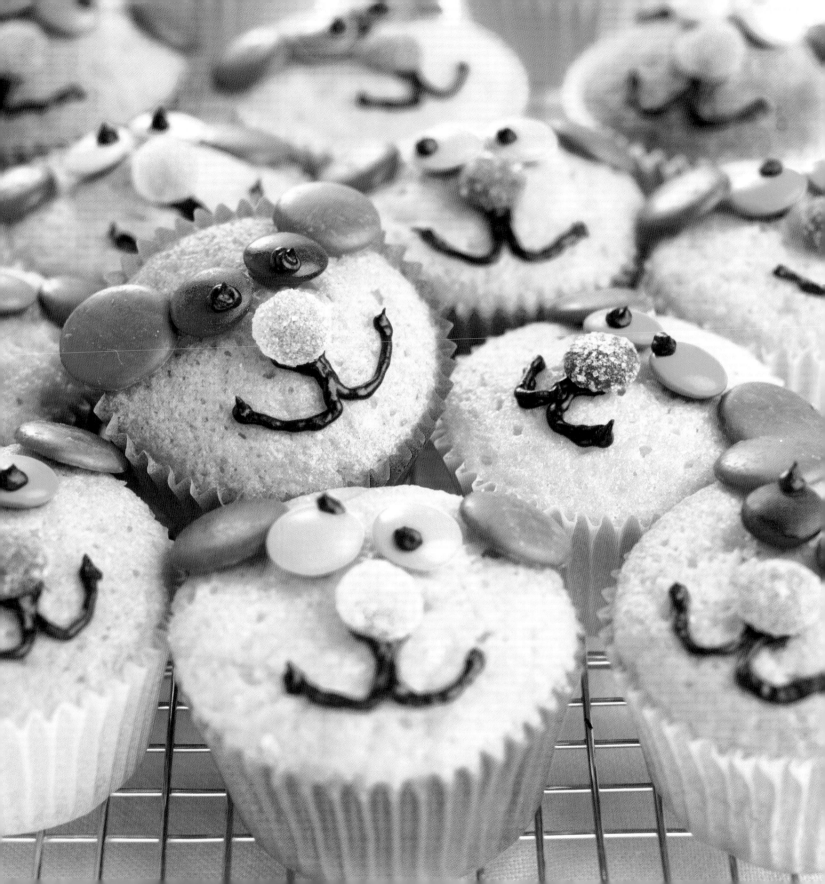

Cranberry and White Chocolate Cookies

These are not to be missed; they are probably my favorite cookies and are so quick and easy to make. You can buy dried cranberries in the supermarket (see photograph).

Makes 20 cookies

1 cup all-purpose flour
½ teaspoon baking soda
½ teaspoon salt
¼ cup ground almonds
¾ cup light brown sugar

1 cup rolled oats
½ cup dried cranberries
1½ ounces white chocolate, cut into chunks
1 stick plus 2 tablespoons unsalted butter
1 large egg yolk or 2 small egg yolks

Preheat the oven to 375°F. Sift together the flour, baking soda, and salt into a large bowl. Stir in the ground almonds, brown sugar, oats, cranberries, and white chocolate chunks.

Melt the butter in a small pan. Stir this into the dry ingredients together with the egg yolk. Mix well, then using your hands, form into walnut-size balls and arrange on two large nonstick baking sheets. Gently press them down to flatten slightly, leaving space between them for the cookies to spread. Bake in the oven for 12 minutes, then remove and allow to cool on a wire rack.

M&M's Cookies

Children will love helping you make these cookies, which are studded with brightly colored candy-coated chocolate. If you find the candy cracks open when baked, you can remove the cookies from the oven and add the extra M&M's on top halfway through baking, so that they are baked in the oven for only 5 minutes (see photograph, page 134).

Makes 20 cookies

½ cup brown sugar
½ cup granulated sugar
2 tablespoons unsalted butter
1 tablespoon vegetable shortening
1 teaspoon pure vanilla extract

1 egg
1¼ cups all-purpose flour
½ teaspoon baking soda
½ teaspoon salt
1 cup chocolate M&M's

Preheat the oven to 350°F. Mix together the sugars, butter, shortening, vanilla, and egg. Sift together the flour, baking soda, and salt and stir into the butter and sugar mixture. Mix in ¾ cup of the M&M's. Using your hands, shape the dough into walnut-size balls and spread well apart on ungreased baking sheets. Flatten slightly and press the remaining M&M's into the dough to decorate the cookies. Bake for about 10 minutes, until lightly golden. The centers will be soft but will firm up later. Allow to cool a little before removing the cookies from the baking sheets and placing them on a wire rack.

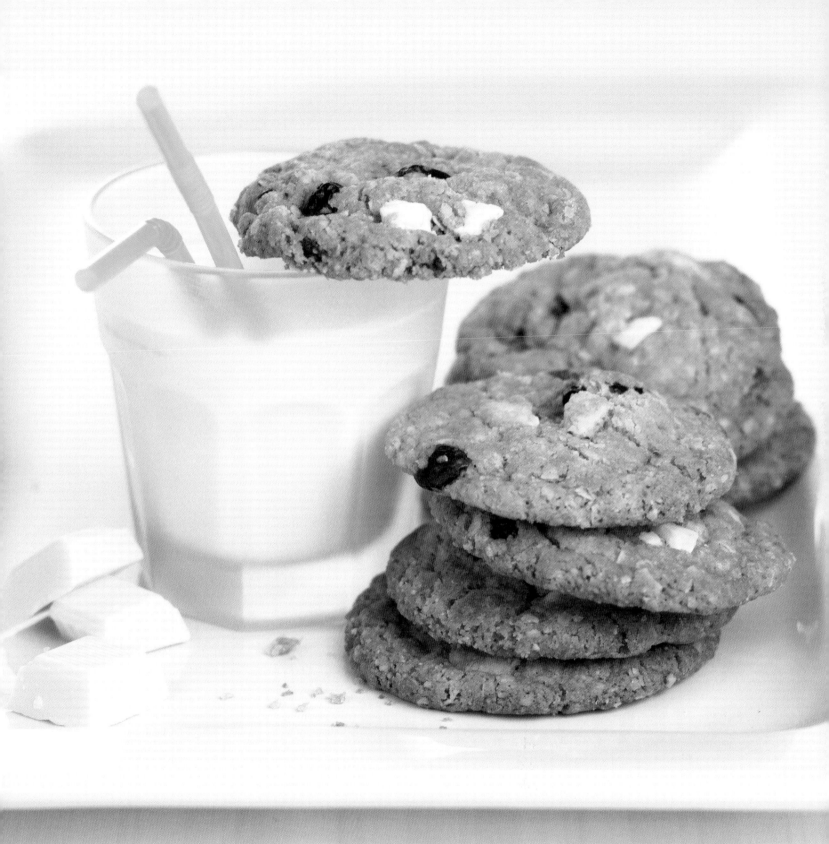

Chocolate-Coffee Cake

This is my favorite chocolate cake recipe. It is lovely and moist with a delicious chocolate flavor, and it keeps really well. Instead of a coffee-flavored buttercream filling, you can make an orange buttercream by leaving out the coffee and using a tablespoon of orange juice and some grated orange zest.
You can decorate the top with candy and novelty candles for a birthday cake.

Makes 8 servings

4½ ounces semisweet chocolate
1½ cups all-purpose flour
1 teaspoon baking soda
¾ cup superfine sugar
⅔ cup light brown sugar
1½ sticks softened unsalted butter
3 eggs
½ cup plus 2 tablespoons heavy cream
1 teaspoon pure vanilla extract

Coffee Buttercream
5½ tablespoons softened unsalted butter
1½ cups confectioners' sugar
½ teaspoon instant coffee dissolved
in 1 teaspoon strong coffee
Confectioners' sugar for dusting

Preheat the oven to 350°F. Grease and line two 8-inch square baking pans. Break the chocolate into pieces and melt in a heatproof bowl over a pan of simmering water and leave to cool.

Sift the flour and baking soda into a large bowl. Beat the sugars together with the butter until smooth. Beat in the eggs one at a time. Add the melted chocolate and beat well. Add the flour to the mixture, alternating with the cream and vanilla, beating after each addition. Divide the mixture between the two prepared pans, smooth the surface with a spatula, and bake for about 25 minutes. Leave the cakes in their pans for a few minutes before placing them on a wire rack to cool.

To make the coffee buttercream, beat together the butter and sugar and then beat in the coffee. Once the cakes are cool, spread the coffee buttercream over the top of one of the cakes and place the other cake on top. Dust with confectioners' sugar.

Coconut Kisses

I defy you to eat only one of these! They're definitely one of my favorites, and your children will enjoy helping you make them as well as eat them.

Makes 25 cookies

1 stick unsalted butter
¼ cup light brown sugar
¼ cup superfine sugar
1 egg, lightly beaten
½ teaspoon pure vanilla extract
½ cup plus 2 tablespoons all-purpose flour

½ teaspoon baking soda
½ teaspoon salt
¾ cup chocolate chips
1½ cups rolled oats
½ cup desiccated coconut

Preheat the oven to 350°F. Cream together the butter and sugars. Add the egg and vanilla. Sift together the flour, baking soda, and salt and beat this into the mixture. Stir in the chocolate chips, oats, and coconut. Form into walnut-size balls, flatten the tops with your hand, and place spaced apart on a lightly greased or lined baking pan. Bake in the oven for 10 to 15 minutes. The cookies will harden when they cool down.

Annabel's Peanut Butter Balls

These scrumptious peanut butter balls are quick and easy to make. They are a good recipe for children to prepare themselves, and you can make them with or without the chocolate coating.

Makes 15 balls

3 tablespoons unsalted butter
½ cup smooth peanut butter
1½ cups Rice Krispies

¾ cup superfine sugar
4 ounces semisweet chocolate, broken into pieces (optional)

Melt the butter and peanut butter in a pan over low heat. Combine the Rice Krispies and sugar in a bowl. Pour the peanut butter mixture into the bowl and stir with a wooden spoon until combined. Using your hands, roll the mixture into about 15 small balls and put them in the refrigerator for about 40 minutes. If making with a chocolate coating, melt the chocolate in a heatproof bowl over a pan of simmering water. Dip the balls halfway into the melted chocolate. Let the chocolate harden; a good way to do this is to balance the balls on an empty ice cube tray.

Carrot and Pineapple Muffins

These are probably my favorite muffins. They are like miniature carrot cakes and are lovely and moist. You can make these with or without the icing.

Makes 12 muffins

¾ cup all-purpose flour
¾ cup whole-wheat flour
1 teaspoon baking powder
¾ teaspoon baking soda
1½ teaspoons ground cinnamon
½ teaspoon salt
¾ cup plus 2 tablespoons vegetable oil
½ cup superfine sugar
2 eggs
¾ cup finely grated carrot

1 cup canned crushed pineapple, drained but with some juice
¾ cup raisins
2 tablespoons chopped pecans (optional)

Cream Cheese Icing
6 ounces cream cheese
¾ cup sifted confectioners' sugar
Half a vanilla bean

Preheat the oven to 350°F. Sift together the flours, baking powder, baking soda, cinnamon, and salt and mix well. In a separate bowl, beat the oil, sugar, and eggs until well blended. Add the grated carrot, crushed pineapple, raisins, and chopped pecans, if using. Gradually add the flour mixture, beating until the ingredients are just combined.

Pour the batter into 12 muffin cups lined with paper liners and bake for 25 minutes. Allow to cool for a few minutes, then remove the muffins from the tin and cool on a wire rack.

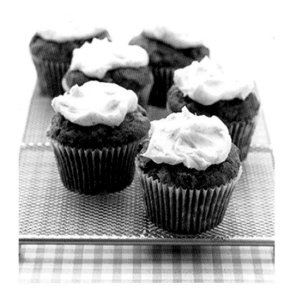

To make the icing, beat the cream cheese together with the confectioners' sugar. Split the vanilla bean and scrape out the tiny black seeds. Stir these into the icing and spread the icing over the tops of the muffins. If you don't have a vanilla bean, you can add a few drops of pure vanilla extract instead.

Zucchini and Raisin Muffins

Here's another good way to get your children to eat vegetables. These muffins are easy to make and taste delicious.

Makes 12 muffins

¾ cup white self-rising flour
1 cup plus 2 tablespoons light brown sugar
½ teaspoon pumpkin pie spice
Pinch of salt
½ teaspoon baking powder
¾ cup whole-grain self-rising flour

¾ cup milk
6 tablespoons melted butter
1½ cups grated zucchini
1 large egg, lightly beaten
¾ cup raisins

Preheat the oven to 350°F. Sift together the white flour, the 1 cup sugar, the pumpkin pie spice, salt, and baking powder. Then sift in the whole-grain flour and save the remaining bran in the sieve.

Mix together the milk, melted butter, zucchini, egg, and raisins. Add the liquid to the flour mixture.

Line a muffin tin with 12 paper liners. Fill each one about two-thirds full. Mix together the reserved bran and the 2 tablespoons brown sugar and sprinkle on top of each muffin. Bake for 25 to 30 minutes.

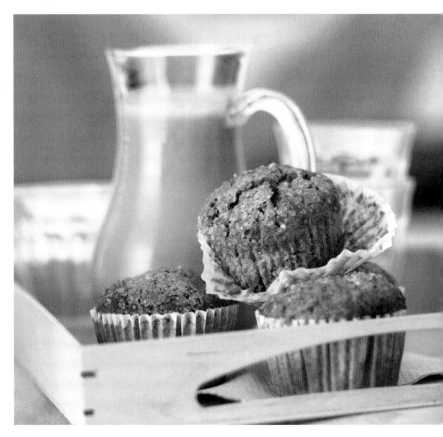

Strawberry Cream Cake

A simple and quick cake to make—and it's sure to be a great favorite with everyone in the family.

Makes 8 servings

6 tablespoons soft margarine
1 cup light brown sugar
3 large eggs
1¼ cups self-rising flour
½ teaspoon grated lemon zest
1 teaspoon pure vanilla extract

Filling / Topping
1 cup heavy cream
3 tablespoons confectioners' sugar
1 pint strawberries, hulled
3 tablespoons strawberry jam

Preheat the oven to 350°F. Grease and line two 8-inch cake pans. Beat together the margarine and sugar, then add the eggs, one at a time, adding 1 tablespoon of flour with the eggs after the first egg to stop the mixture from curdling. Beat in the remaining flour, the lemon zest, vanilla, and 1 tablespoon of water until light and fluffy.

Divide the mixture between the prepared pans and bake in the oven for about 20 minutes or until lightly golden and risen. Allow to cool a little and then turn them out of the pans and put on a wire rack to cool.

Whip the cream with the sugar until firm. Thinly slice two-thirds of the strawberries. Stir the strawberries into two-thirds of the whipped cream. Spread the strawberry jam over one of the layers, top with the strawberries-and-cream mixture, and place the other layer on top. Using the remaining whipped cream, pipe rosettes around the edge of the cake and place half a strawberry on top of each rosette. Keep refrigerated until ready to serve.

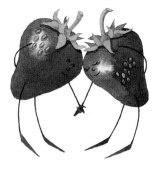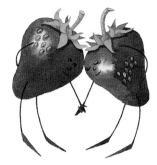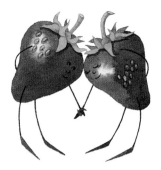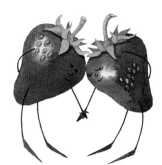

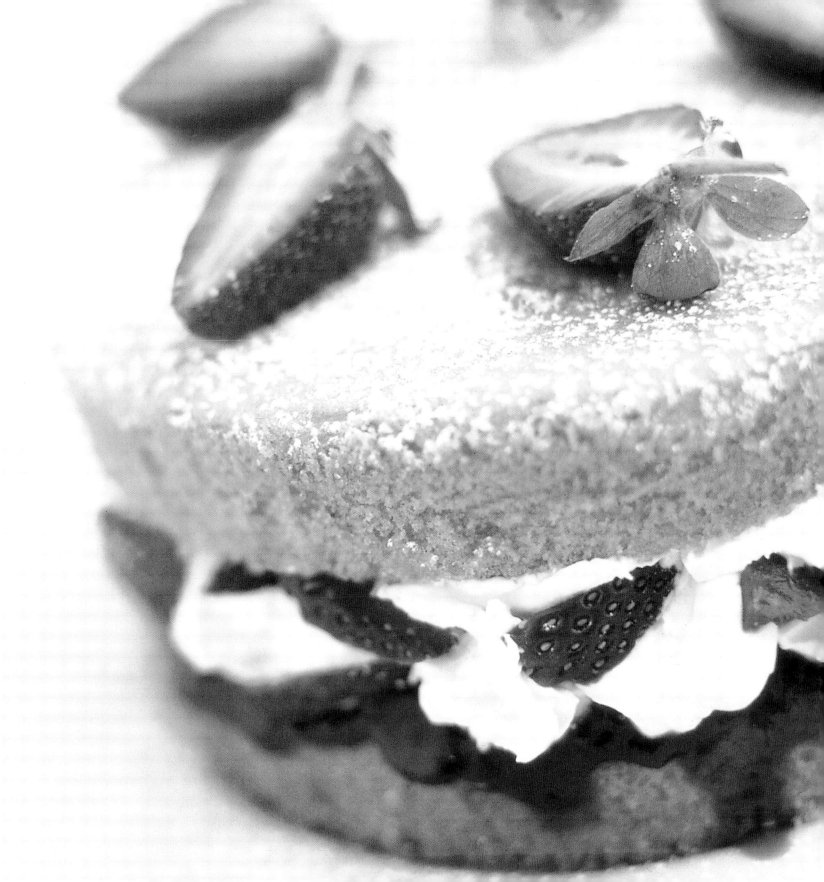

Apple Smiles

This snack is easy to prepare and will certainly bring a smile to your child's face! For a healthier variation, use small cubes of cheese instead of mini-marshmallows (see photograph).

Makes 4 apple smiles

Smooth peanut butter
1 red apple, cored and sliced into eighths

Squeeze of lemon juice
Miniature marshmallows

Spread peanut butter on one side of each apple slice (squeeze a little lemon juice over the apple if not serving immediately). Place four miniature marshmallows on one apple slice and then lay another apple slice, peanut butter side down, on top.

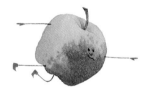 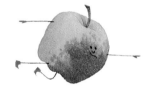 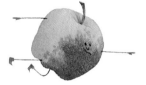

Divinely Decadent Fruity Dark Chocolate Bars

These no-bake chocolate fruit-and-nut bars are amazingly good and one of my favorite treats. Indulge yourself and make sure they're hidden when Daddy or Mommy comes home. They are also fun for children to make themselves.

Makes 12 bars

8 ounces bittersweet chocolate
6 tablespoons unsalted butter
One 14-ounce can of condensed milk
8 ounces graham crackers, broken into pieces

4 ounces dried apricots, roughly chopped
¼ cup raisins
¼ cup roughly chopped pecans

Break the chocolate into squares and cut the butter into pieces, put these into a bowl, and microwave on full power for about 3 minutes, stirring halfway through. (Alternatively, the chocolate and butter can be melted in a bowl over a saucepan of simmering water.) Stir the condensed milk into the chocolate mixture and mix in the broken graham crackers, chopped apricots, raisins, and chopped pecans. Line an 11 x 7-inch shallow cake pan with clear plastic, allowing the sides to overhang. Spoon the mixture into the pan and press down, but still leave the top a little rough. Place in the refrigerator to set. Once set, lift out of the pan by the overhanging clear plastic and cut into small bars. Keep chilled in the refrigerator.

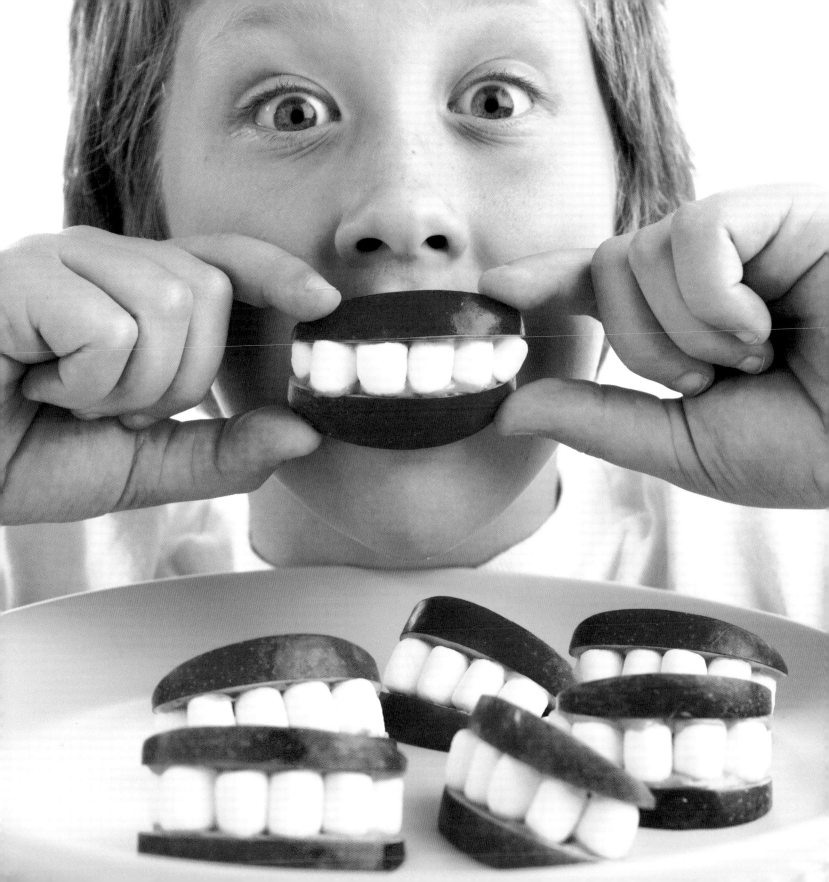

Glossy Dark and White Chocolate Brownies

Two chocolates are combined to make these irresistible squares of rich, chewy brownies (see photograph).

Makes 16 squares

5 ounces dark chocolate (semisweet or bittersweet), chopped
6 tablespoons unsalted butter
1 teaspoon pure vanilla extract
1 cup superfine sugar
2 eggs
1 egg yolk
⅔ cup all-purpose flour

¼ teaspoon salt
1 cup white chocolate morsels or chopped white chocolate

Chocolate Satin Glaze
3 ounces dark chocolate, chopped
1 tablespoon unsalted butter
½ cup white chocolate morsels

Preheat the oven to 350°F and grease and line an 8-inch square baking pan. Put the dark chocolate and butter into a bowl and microwave for 2 minutes on high (or melt in a saucepan over gentle heat, stirring constantly). Stir in the vanilla and sugar, then add the eggs and yolk, one at a time, stirring after each addition. Sift together the flour and salt and mix this into the chocolate mixture with the white chocolate morsels. Pour the batter into the prepared pan and bake in the oven for about 30 minutes.

To prepare the glaze, melt the dark chocolate and butter together and spread over the cooled brownies. Melt the white chocolate morsels, and using a teaspoon, trail 5 lines horizontally across the brownies about ½ inch apart. With a blunt knife draw vertical lines lightly through the chocolate glaze to create a pattern. Cut into 16 squares.

Mars Bars and Rice Krispies Slices

These are very popular for parties and no one will know what they are made of if you don't tell them! They will keep for one week if they are not gobbled up sooner!

Makes 20 slices

Three 1½-ounce Mars Bars
6 tablespoons unsalted butter
1 cup Rice Krispies

Topping
7 ounces chocolate (milk or semisweet)
2 tablespoons unsalted butter

Grease a 9-inch square pan. Melt the Mars Bars and butter in a saucepan, stirring occasionally (do not boil). Stir in the Rice Krispies. Press into the pan and set aside in the refrigerator to set for about 1 hour. For the topping, put the chocolate and butter in a saucepan and heat gently, stirring occasionally, until melted. Spread the topping over the Rice Krispies mixture and, when cool, put in the refrigerator to set. With a sharp knife, cut into 20 slices.

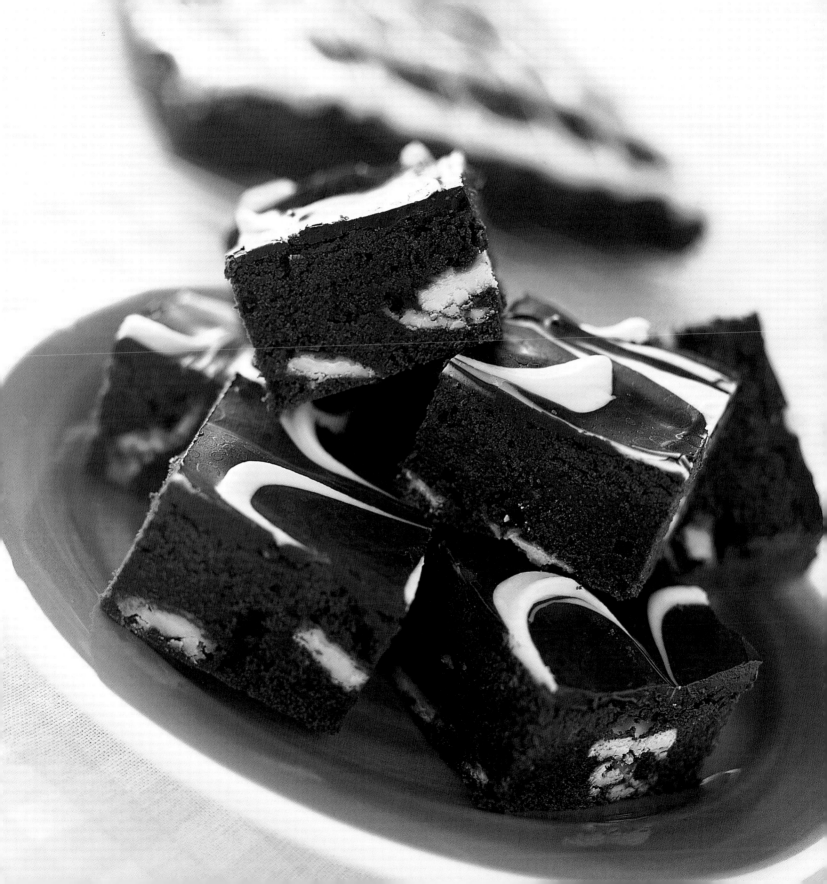

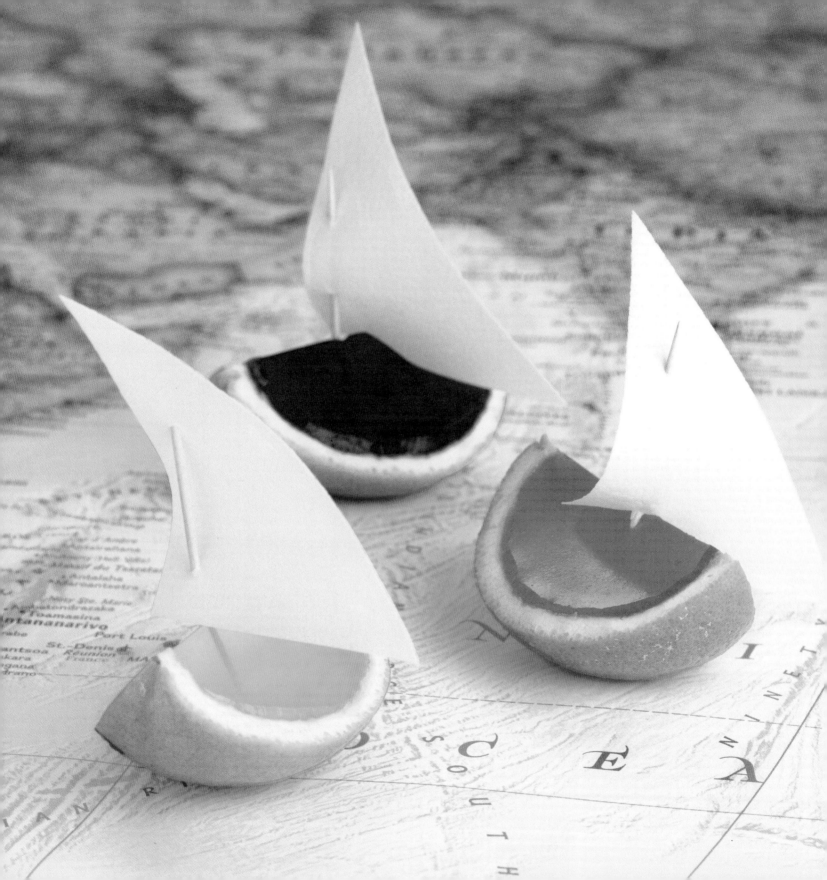

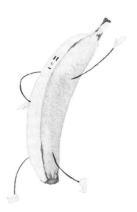

Desserts

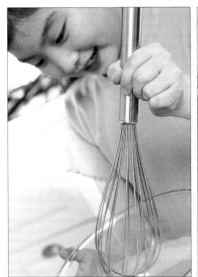

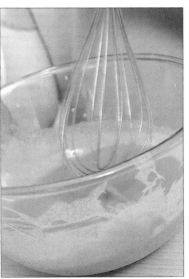

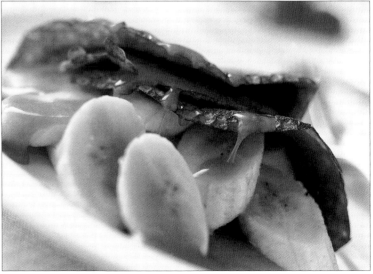

Caramelized Almond Ice Cream

This ice cream tastes sensational, is very simple to make, and you don't need to use an ice cream machine. It is also very good with pecans instead of almonds. It goes well with fresh peaches, which can be served hot with some ice cream on the side. Simply wash, peel, and pit the peaches, and sprinkle with a little brown sugar. Place under a preheated broiler for a few minutes.

Makes 6 servings

One 12-ounce can of evaporated milk

Caramelized Almonds
1¾ cups blanched almonds
1¾ cups light brown sugar

3 tablespoons cold water

1 cup superfine sugar
1 cup heavy cream
2 teaspoons pure vanilla extract

Chill the can of evaporated milk in the freezer for about 3 hours. For the caramelized almonds, toast the almonds under a preheated broiler for a few minutes until golden, turning once. Put the sugar into a heavy-bottomed saucepan together with the water and cook, stirring, over low heat until it caramelizes. Stir in the almonds and coat with the sticky caramel. Transfer to a baking tray to cool down.

Once cool, place the caramelized almonds in a kitchen towel, wrap them up, and crush with a mallet or rolling pin. Whip the frozen milk with the superfine sugar until thick. Whip the cream and mix into the evaporated milk mixture together with the vanilla and the crushed almonds. Put into a suitable container and freeze.

Summer Fruit Brûlée with Amaretto Cookies

This is one of my favorite desserts and is particularly good in summer when peaches and berry fruits are in season. You can also make this using other combinations of fruits, but it's important that the fruit be really ripe and have a good flavor. Fruits that work well are mangoes, grapes, nectarines, strawberries, and kiwis, and you could mix in some passion fruit pulp if you like.

Makes 6 servings

1 cup blueberries
1 cup raspberries
2 ripe juicy peaches, peeled, pitted, and chopped

12 amaretto cookies, crushed
1 cup crème fraîche or a mixture of plain yogurt and heavy cream

Mix the fruit together and arrange in an ovenproof dish. Sprinkle with the crushed amaretto cookies and top with the crème fraîche. Chill in the refrigerator for at least 1 hour. Sprinkle with the brown sugar and place under a preheated broiler for a few minutes, until golden.

Louise's Apple and Blackberry Pudding

Louise is a good friend of mine who has two children, Olivia and Ben, both of whom are very fussy eaters. This is one of her children's favorite desserts, and it's quick and easy to make. Blackberries are rich in vitamin C, and my children love them. Here the slightly tart flavor of the fruit blends really well with the almond topping. Serve hot on its own or with custard or vanilla ice cream.

Makes 4 servings

1 stick unsalted butter
1 cup superfine sugar
2 eggs
¾ cup ground almonds

1 teaspoon almond extract
1 pound cooking apples, cored, peeled, and sliced
2 cups (1 pint) blackberries, fresh or frozen

Preheat the oven to 325°F. Cream together the butter and sugar, then beat in the eggs, ground almonds, and almond extract. Combine the apples and blackberries and place in an ovenproof dish. Spread the topping over the fruit and bake in the oven for 45 minutes.

Simple Berry Fruit Brûlée

Berries, with their high antioxidant levels, are some of the most delicious and powerful disease-fighting foods available. All berries are rich in vitamin C, but strawberries contain more than any other berry. Blueberries are a true superfood and have the highest antioxidant properties of all fruits.

Makes 4 servings

2 cups (1 pint) mixed fresh berries: blueberries, strawberries, raspberries, blackberries
⅔ cup heavy cream
¾ cup plain yogurt

2 tablespoons confectioners' sugar
½ teaspoon pure vanilla extract
1½ tablespoons light brown sugar

Divide the berries among 4 small (4-inch diameter) ramekins or heatproof glass dishes. Lightly whip the cream until it forms soft peaks. Fold in the yogurt, confectioners' sugar, and vanilla. Spoon the yogurt mixture over the fruit. Sprinkle with the light brown sugar and place under a preheated broiler for 2 to 3 minutes, until golden and bubbling.

Desert Island Pineapple

Here is a very attractive way to serve fresh fruit for a special occasion (see photograph).

**Makes 6
servings**

*1 large pineapple
Assorted fruit, such as strawberries,
blueberries, and raspberries*

White grapes

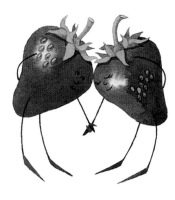

Choose a large pineapple with attractive-looking leaves. Cut the base flat and peel the pineapple, leaving some peel and flesh at the bottom to make a steady base for the tree. With a sharp knife, remove the rest of the flesh, leaving the hard core to form the trunk of the tree.

Place the palm tree on a flat plate and arrange the chunks of pineapple around it together with the assorted fresh fruit, and decorate the palm tree with the white grapes; small bunches can be tied to the tree with a length of string.

Fresh Fruit Pops

If there is one food that almost no child can resist, it has to be an ice pop, so why not make a healthy version using fresh fruit? You can also make delicious pops by simply freezing pure fruit juice or fruit smoothies in an ice pop mold.

Makes 6 pops

*¼ cup superfine sugar
¼ cup water
1¼ cups halved strawberries*

*1 cup raspberries
1 large ripe peach, pitted, peeled, and diced
Juice of 2 medium oranges*

Put the sugar and water into a small saucepan, bring to a boil, and stir until the sugar has dissolved. Puree the strawberries, raspberries, and peach in a blender and strain to remove the seeds. Combine the fruit puree with the orange juice and sugar syrup. Pour into an ice pop mold and freeze.

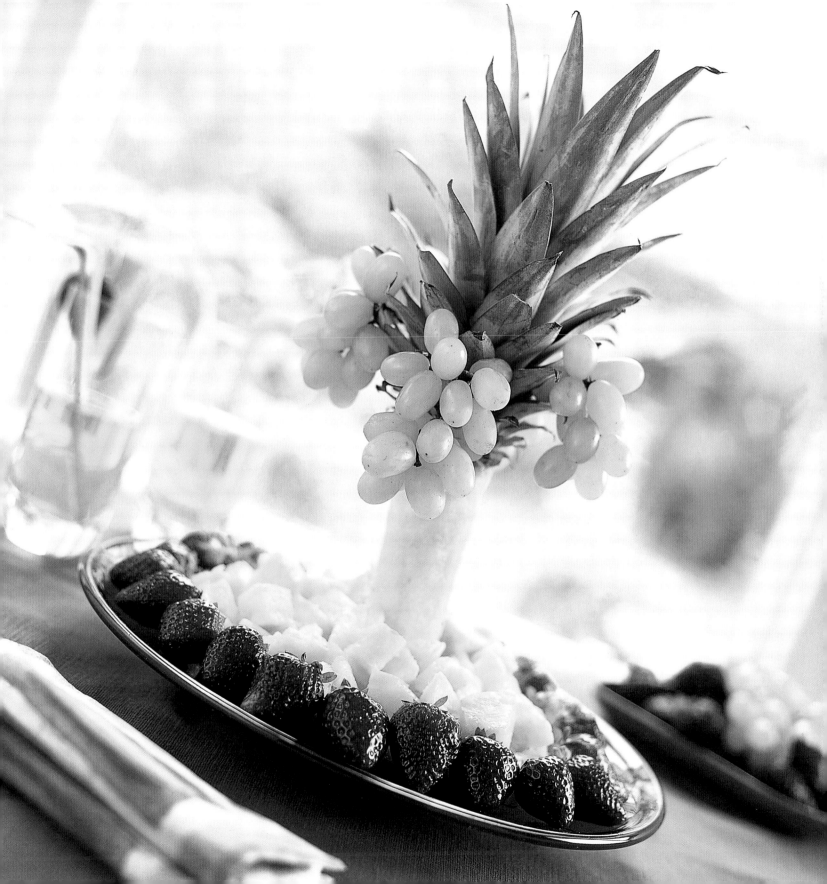

Auntie Ruthie's Quick and Easy Cheesecake

It will be hard to beat the taste of this delicious cheesecake, and it's very quick and simple to prepare. Serve it plain or with the fresh strawberry topping. For best results use a good-quality fresh cream cheese.

Makes 6 servings

8 ounces graham crackers
1 stick plus 2 tablespoons unsalted butter
1½ pounds cream cheese
1¼ cups superfine sugar
2 large eggs
1 teaspoon pure vanilla extract
2 cups sour cream
2 tablespoons granulated sugar

Strawberry Topping

3 tablespoons seedless raspberry jam
2 pints strawberries, hulled and cut in half

Preheat the oven to 350°F. To make the base, crush the graham crackers. This can be done by breaking them up, putting them in a plastic bag, and crushing them with a rolling pin. Or you can break them up in a food processor. Melt the butter and stir in the crumbs.

Grease and line a 9-inch springform pan and spoon the crumbs over the bottom, pressing down well (a potato masher is useful for this). In a food processor, beat together the cream cheese, sugar, eggs, vanilla, and 1 cup of the sour cream. Pour the cream cheese mixture over the crumb base and bake in the oven for 25 minutes. Top with the remaining 1 cup sour cream mixed with the granulated sugar and then bake for 15 minutes more.

While the cake is baking in the oven, you can prepare the topping. Spread the raspberry jam in a baking dish and arrange half the strawberries on top. Cover with foil and put in the oven for 20 minutes. Strain the sauce and discard the cooked strawberries. Simmer the sauce in a small saucepan until syrupy. Arrange the remaining strawberries on top of the cake and brush with the syrup.

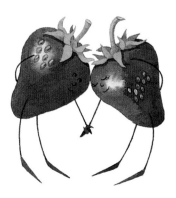

Tiramisù

This popular Italian dessert, which means "pick me up," is quick and easy to make and is a great way to end a meal. Since this dessert contains raw eggs, it should not be eaten by young children.

Makes 6 servings

3 eggs
1 cup superfine sugar
3½ tablespoons marsala wine
14 ounces mascarpone cheese

Pinch of salt
1 cup strong coffee
24 ladyfingers
1 tablespoon cocoa powder

Separate the eggs, putting the yolks into one mixing bowl and 2 of the egg whites into another bowl (discard the remaining white). Add the sugar to the egg yolks and beat until thick and creamy. Stir in the marsala and the mascarpone cheese and mix together with the beaten yolks. Add a pinch of salt to the egg whites and beat until they form stiff peaks. Fold the egg whites into the mascarpone mixture until combined. Choose a rectangular dish in which to serve the tiramisù or prepare individual portions in small dessert bowls. Pour the coffee into a shallow bowl and dip the ladyfingers into the coffee one at a time so that they absorb some of the liquid.

Arrange 12 of the ladyfingers in the bottom of the dish, cover with half the mascarpone mixture, arrange the remaining 12 ladyfingers, then spoon the remaining mascarpone mixture on top. Sprinkle the surface with the cocoa powder; this is best done using a sieve. Chill in the refrigerator for about 4 hours before serving.

Gelatin Boats

These are one of the most popular party foods that I make (see photograph, page 156).

Makes 16 boats

4 large oranges, halved
Two 4½-ounce packages of flavored gelatin,
such as raspberry, strawberry, peach, orange,
and lime

4 sheets of rice paper
16 toothpicks

With a sharp knife, remove the inside flesh of the oranges and carefully scrape out the membrane, taking care not to make a hole in the skin of the oranges. Prepare the gelatin, but follow the instructions using only half the amount of water, as you will need a more concentrated gelatin to hold its shape. Fill each of the hollow orange halves with gelatin right to the top. If you like, you can place them in muffin tins to keep them steady. Refrigerate until set and then trim the orange halves so that the skin of the orange is level with the gelatin. Cut the oranges in half again with a sharp knife. Cut 16 triangles out of the rice paper and secure with the toothpicks to make sails.

Chocolate Banana Pancakes

My son, Nicholas, loves these. He likes to spread the sauce over the pancakes and then roll them up like a jelly roll. These pancakes are also good with fresh orange segments or raspberries as well as the sliced bananas.

Makes 8 pancakes

³/₄ cup all-purpose flour
¼ teaspoon salt
1 tablespoon cocoa powder
1 tablespoon superfine sugar
2 eggs, lightly beaten
¾ cup milk
¼ cup water
2 tablespoons melted butter,
plus extra for frying
A little grated orange zest (optional)

Toffee Sauce
4 tablespoons unsalted butter
½ cup light brown sugar
¼ cup heavy cream
2 tablespoons corn syrup or golden syrup

4 small bananas, sliced, or 2 bananas and some orange segments or fresh raspberries

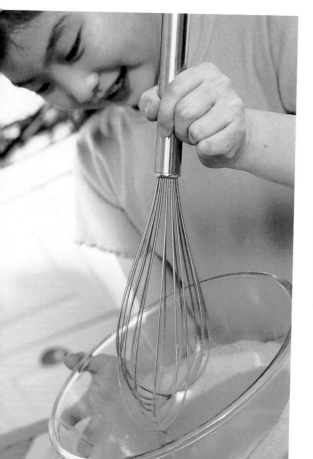

Sift the flour, salt, cocoa powder, and sugar into a bowl. Make a well in the center and add the eggs and ¼ cup plus 2 tablespoons of the milk. Using a whisk, beat together the ingredients until smooth. Whisk in the remaining milk and the water to make a smooth batter, then stir in the butter and orange zest, if using. This can be set aside in the refrigerator for up to 30 minutes if you like.

To make the pancakes, brush a heavy 7- or 8-inch frying pan with melted butter and when hot, ladle in some of the batter and swirl around the frying pan to form a thin layer. Cook for a minute or so on each side.

To make the toffee sauce, place the butter, sugar, cream, and syrup in a pan. Heat gently until melted, then bring to a boil and let bubble for 1 minute. Spoon the fruit onto one side of the pancake, drizzle with some of the sauce, fold the pancake in half and then in quarters, and spoon on some more of the toffee sauce.

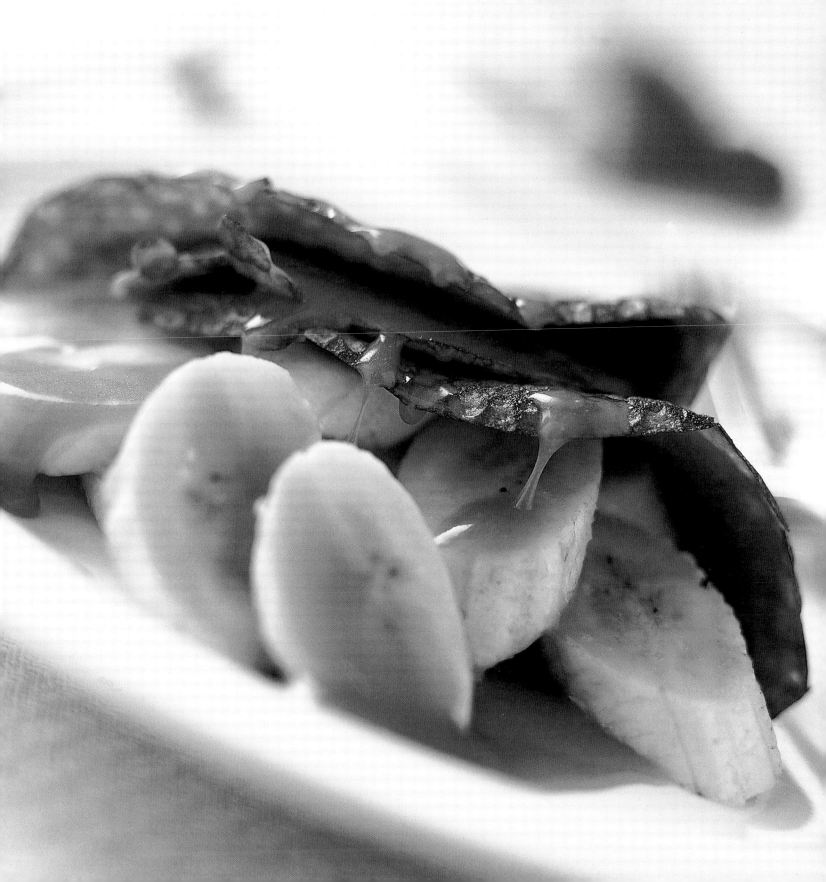

Evelyn's Noodle Pudding

This is a favorite dessert that my mother used to make when I was a child. I now make it for my son, Nicholas, who loves it just as much as I did, if not more so.

Makes 6 servings

Butter
8 ounces vermicelli
2 eggs
3 tablespoons heavy cream
3 tablespoons superfine sugar

¾ teaspoon pure vanilla extract
¾ cup each dark raisins and golden raisins
1 teaspoon ground cinnamon
2 teaspoons brown sugar

Preheat the oven to 350°F. Thoroughly butter a fairly shallow 12- by 8-inch ovenproof dish. Cook the vermicelli in a large pot of lightly salted boiling water according to the instructions on the package. When cooked, rinse under cold water. Beat the eggs well in a large bowl, then add the cream, sugar, vanilla, raisins, and cinnamon. Fold in the vermicelli and pour into the prepared dish. Sprinkle with the brown sugar and dot the top with a little butter. Bake in the oven for 35 minutes.

Apple, Nectarine, and Raspberry Crumble

A really good crumble bursting with fruit is comfort food at its very best. Other good fruit fillings are rhubarb, gooseberry, blackberry, and apple or strawberry and plum. Serve hot with vanilla ice cream or custard.

Makes 5 servings

2 sweet eating apples
2 tablespoons unsalted butter
2 tablespoons light brown sugar
2 white nectarines or peaches
1½ cups raspberries
3 tablespoons ground almonds

Topping
1 cup all-purpose flour
Generous pinch of salt
½ cup light brown sugar
1 stick cold unsalted butter, cut into pieces
½ cup ground almonds

Preheat the oven to 400°F. Peel and core the apples and cut into slices. Melt the butter in a saucepan. Add the sliced apples to the pan, sprinkle with the sugar, and cook for 2 to 3 minutes. Remove from the heat. Peel and pit the nectarines or peaches and cut into slices. Add these to the cooked apples together with the raspberries. Sprinkle the ground almonds into a suitable ovenproof dish (a round dish with a 7-inch diameter is ideal). Spoon the fruit into the dish. To make the topping, mix the flour with the salt and sugar. Cut the butter into pieces and rub in with your fingertips until the mixture resembles bread crumbs. Rub in the ground almonds and cover the fruit with the crumble topping. Sprinkle with a tablespoon of water, which will help to make the topping crispy. Bake in the oven for 30 to 35 minutes or until the topping is lightly golden.

Iced Berries with Hot White Chocolate Sauce

The slightly frozen berries melt into the warm chocolate sauce, giving a delicious contrast.

Makes 4 servings

1 pound mixed berries, such as blackberries, blueberries, raspberries, and red currants

Sauce
5 ounces white chocolate
½ cup heavy cream

Put the berries in a suitable container and place in the freezer for a couple of hours, until semifrozen. Melt the white chocolate in the cream in a heatproof bowl over a pan of simmering water. Don't allow the base of the bowl to come into contact with the water. Stir until the chocolate has melted into the cream. Scatter the semifrozen berries on 4 plates or in shallow bowls, pour on the hot chocolate sauce, and serve immediately.

Yvonne's Malva Pudding

Yvonne is a very good friend of mine who lives in Cape Town. I used to teach her daughter to play the harp, and whenever I gave concerts, Yvonne would present me with a cookbook instead of a bouquet of flowers. She is the most fantastic cook, and we used to swap recipes long before I ever thought of writing cookbooks myself.

Makes 8 servings

Sponge Pudding
1½ cups sifted all-purpose flour
1 egg, lightly beaten
1½ teaspoons baking soda
1 teaspoon white vinegar
1 cup superfine sugar
1 cup milk
Pinch of salt
1 heaping tablespoon apricot jam
1 tablespoon unsalted butter

Sauce
1½ cups superfine sugar
1 cup milk
1 cup heavy cream
2 tablespoons unsalted butter
1 teaspoon pure vanilla extract

Preheat the oven to 350°F. Grease an ovenproof dish that measures approximately 10 by 8 inches. Combine the ingredients for the pudding to form a smooth batter. Pour into the prepared dish and bake for 35 minutes or until a knife comes out clean. Combine all the ingredients for the sauce in a pan, stir over medium heat, and bring just to a boil, but do not let boil. Make several holes in the top of the pudding with a skewer and pour half the sauce over the pudding and into the holes. Serve with the remaining sauce on the side.

Nicholas's Dream Dessert

My son, Nicholas, and I concocted this heavenly dessert together. We decided to design a dessert using fresh summer berries, cream, and crushed meringue. It was a huge success with the whole family and there was not a scrap left. This is also an easy and fun recipe to make with your child (see photograph).

Makes 6 servings

2 pints raspberries
3 to 4 tablespoons superfine sugar
1½ cups quartered strawberries

1 cup heavy cream
Few drops of pure vanilla extract
4 ready-made meringues

Put half the raspberries into a saucepan and heat gently until they become mushy. Press the raspberries through a sieve and reserve the sauce in a small saucepan. Add the sugar to taste and stir over low heat until the sugar is dissolved. Stir the remaining raspberries and the strawberries into the sauce.

Whip the cream together with the vanilla until stiff but not too thick. Break the meringues into pieces and fold these into the whipped cream. Spoon a little of the cream-and-meringue mixture into each of 6 parfait glasses, cover with some of the berries, and then repeat each layer and top with a sprig of mint, some crushed meringue, or some additional raspberries.

Berried Treasure

You can buy rose water in many supermarkets, and it gives this fruit compote a lovely flavor. The pomegranate seeds add a crunchy texture that complements the berry fruits.

Makes 4 servings

2 peaches
1 tablespoon unsalted butter
2 tablespoons superfine sugar
1 tablespoon rose water
1 cup strawberries

1 cup blackberries
1 cup blueberries
1 cup raspberries
½ pomegranate (optional)

Halve and pit the peaches, and cut each half into four slices. Melt the butter in a heavy-bottomed saucepan and sauté the peaches for 1 minute. Sprinkle with the sugar and cook for 1 minute more. Add the rose water, strawberries, blackberries, and blueberries, and heat for about 1 minute. Remove from the heat and stir in the raspberries and pomegranate seeds, if using.

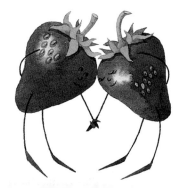

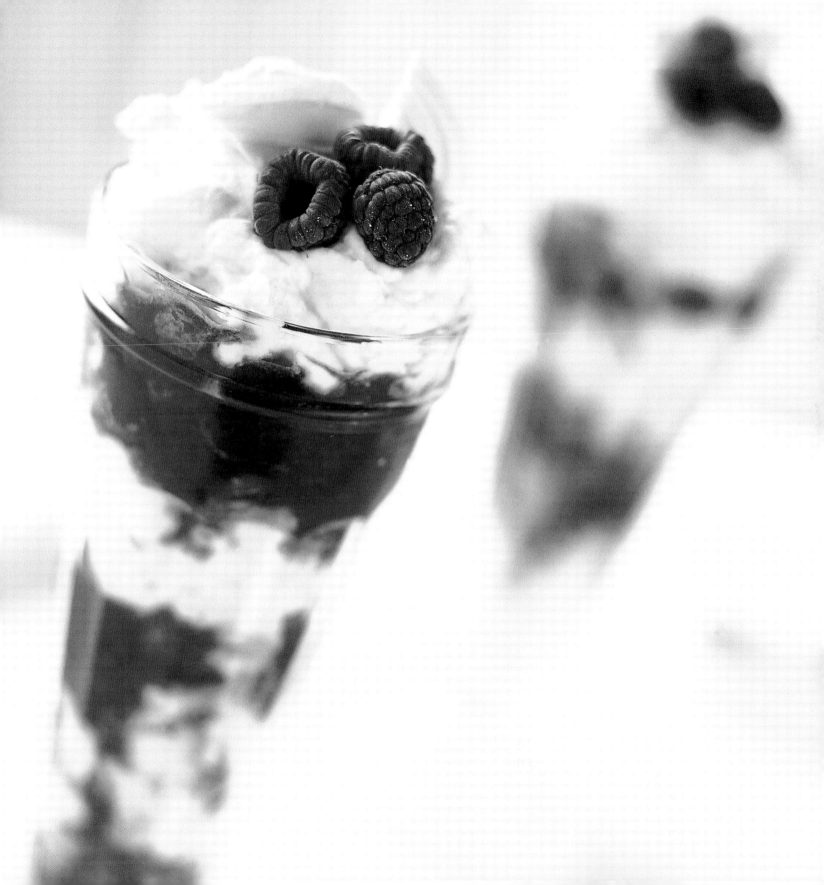

Index

Acknowledgments

I want to thank all the children and parents who have been guinea pigs to the successes and failures of my culinary experiments. In particular my mother, Evelyn Etkind, who very seldom uses her own kitchen but has hosted many dinner parties by raiding the contents of my fridge after a day's recipe testing; and my children, Nicholas, Lara, and Scarlett, and their many friends, who have eaten their way through all the recipes in this book and enjoyed lending a hand in cooking some, too. Also my husband, Simon, who will be pleased to sit down to dinner in peace without having me ask "Well, what do you think?" before being given the chance to swallow the first mouthful.

I would also like to thank Amelia Thorpe, Joanna Carreras, Carey Smith, Sarah Lavelle, Emma Callery, Christine Carter, Alison Shackleton, Dave King, Daniel Pangbourne, Harry Ormesher, Val Barrett, Tessa Evelegh, David Karmel, Jacqui Morley, Marina Magpoc, Letty Catada, Nadine Wickenden, Jane Hamilton, Mary Jones, Judith Curr, Tim Shaw, Greer Hendricks, Suzanne O'Neill, Justin Loeber, Caitlin Friedman, and Aimee Bianca.

About the Author

ANNABEL KARMEL is a leading author on cooking for children. After the tragic loss of her first child, who died of a rare viral disease at just three months, Annabel wrote her first book, *The Healthy Baby Meal Planner* (Simon & Schuster), which is now an international bestseller and the leading book on feeding young children. Annabel has written twelve more bestselling books on feeding children, including *First Meals, Superfoods for Babies and Children, Lunchboxes, The Mom and Me Cookbook,* and *The Complete First Year Planner.* She is a pioneering food writer and an expert in devising tasty, nutritious, and innovative meals for children without the need for parents to spend hours in the kitchen.

Children are exacting critics, and while they are rarely interested in whether their food is healthy, they do care if it tastes good. Accordingly, all of Annabel's recipes are tested on a panel of children to make sure that they have that magical ingredient—child appeal.

Annabel appears regularly on TV in the UK. Her latest appearance was on the "Foodie Godmother" series, which was an eight-part series shown on the UK's most popular daytime talk show, *Richard and Judy.* In this series, Annabel traveled around England helping to solve the eating problems of ultrafussy eaters. She has also appeared on many TV programs in the United States, including *Today, Good Day New York,* and the *CBS Early Show,* and she travels frequently to the States.

Annabel lives in London and has three children, Nicholas, Lara, and Scarlett. She designed the Marks & Spencer food line for children in the UK and is launching her own line of healthy frozen meals for young children in 2006. She is also launching a complete line of equipment for making baby food. She has an extensive website on feeding and looking after children—visit www.annabelkarmel.com—and is also Celebrity Chef on the BBC website www.bbc.co.uk/food.